Bedtime Wordsearch

Bedtime Wordsearch

Puzzles To help you relax before you go to sleep

This edition published in 2020 by Arcturus Publishing Limited
26/27 Bickels Yard, 151–153 Bermondsey Street,
London SE1 3HA

AD008162NT

Printed in the US

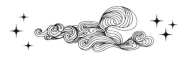

INTRODUCTION

Sleep problems are so common that reportedly up to 30% of adults suffer from some sort of disrupted sleep. But there are many things we can do to help us sleep more soundly.

"The feeling of sleepiness when you are not in bed, and can't get there, is the meanest feeling in the world."
Edgar Watson Howe

What is sleep?
Sleep is the naturally occurring, altered state of consciousness that affects the body and mind. The nervous system becomes relatively inactive, muscle activity is reduced, and the eyes are closed. This may lead us to believe that it is a time when our minds and bodies completely shut down, but this is not the case.

Why does sleep matter?
It is perhaps surprising to learn that the reasons that we sleep are still not fully understood but we do know that good sleep is vital to our wellbeing. During the day our brains take in a huge amount of information. This is not immediately processed but is stored in our short-term memory; it is during sleep that this information is processed, or consolidated, moving to our long-term memory. It is also a time of healing and rejuvenation for our cells and bodies. So, though we may not fully understand sleep, we do know that it plays a key role in keeping us healthy both mentally and physically.

"For sleep, one needs endless depths of blackness to sink into; daylight is too shallow, it will not cover one."
Anne Morrow Lindbergh

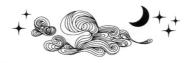

How can I improve my sleep?

Though there can be underlying medical causes to sleep problems which may need addressing there are some easy ways to try to improve your sleep. Monitoring your habits, including sleep times, diet, and exercise can help; an awareness of our habits can help us to understand our body's needs. Sleep can also be improved by establishing and sticking to a bedtime routine, and this is where the relaxing puzzles in this collection can help.

How can puzzles help?

A bedtime routine can include self-care rituals, meditation, switching off from technology, and relaxing activities. One such activity is the completion of puzzles, which have proven mindfulness benefits in helping us to switch off. By concentrating only on the puzzle, we can forget the troubles and cares of the day, clearing our mind for sleep.

In this book you will find small wordsearch puzzles for a quick bedtime activity, as well as full-sized puzzles for when you need longer to unwind. Many of the puzzles are themed in a sleep-related way and each is accompanied by a sleep-related quote, fact, or tip, or an interpretation of a common dream symbol based on the pioneering work of Pamela Ball. Also interspersed throughout are sleep exercises that can be used to assess and improve your sleep. And before you know it you'll be ready for a sound sleep.

"Goodnight room. Goodnight moon. Goodnight cow jumping over the moon. Goodnight light, and the red balloon..."
Margaret Wise Brown

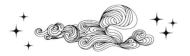

1 Peace

ACCORD
GOODWILL
HARMONY
LOVE
QUIET

RECONCILE
RESOLVE
TRANQUIL
TRUCE
UNITY

```
G N L E V O L R E
O D I P I Y I E C
O T U U T T A C H
D E Q I G C E O A
W I N R C C S N R
I U A O U R I C M
L Q R R H E N I O
L D T I A G E L N
E V L O S E R E Y
```

2 Joy

BLISS
CHEER
DELIGHT
ECSTASY
ELATION

GLAD
GLEE
HAPPINESS
MERRY
THRILL

```
A T U B D R B Y H
N H F A M L S A D
O F L Y I A P Y E
I G F S T P T F L
T L S S I D M R I
A N C N B R E E G
L E E L G N R E H
E S P L L I R H T
S I V E T O Y C B
```

"Sleep in peace, and wake in joy."

William Shakespeare

Nocturnal Creatures

```
U E R E T A R E B H R A A
I T A R K C A L B B E N L
M C B O S S K O F Y G E L
C R M A C L R N L F D Y I
P I G T S O O S U I A H H
A C Y A M R E W N K B F C
N K B B H E T G L M S P N
G E U M E T O O H O E N I
O T V O A S E O L N R C H
L O C W J M T Y E E L I C
I Y A G R A M I A S C I S
N O P B S H K V S E E O M
S C O R P I O N T E Y D L
F B G T T O O C I D N A B
U T A R I N A D E K C A H
```

AYE-AYE   CRICKET   OCELOT
BADGER   DINGO   PANGOLIN
BANDICOOT   HAMSTER   SCORPION
BLACK RAT   HYENA   SKUNK
CHINCHILLA   KINKAJOU   SLOW LORIS
COYOTE   MARGAY   WOMBAT

In our dreams—Animals:

Animals can represent intuitive natural emotions and actions we may be repressing, consider the particular animal and their natural traits to understand.

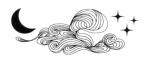

Can't Sleep

```
I  T  R  E  Y  E  D  E  R  S  E  T  H
F  V  D  S  W  I  D  E  A  W  A  K  E
P  G  D  E  A  S  Y  S  W  O  R  D  D
Y  V  P  E  C  N  G  I  V  R  S  O  B
V  P  V  O  I  O  X  W  E  C  T  G  S
L  E  T  H  A  R  G  I  C  U  R  N  K
G  I  I  Y  C  I  R  L  O  O  E  I  N
A  F  S  I  A  N  N  O  D  U  S  K  I
L  S  C  T  N  G  L  T  W  D  S  N  W
T  R  H  A  L  S  I  R  H  E  E  I  Y
E  D  W  U  A  E  O  T  H  R  D  H  T
J  L  B  S  T  T  S  M  A  I  H  T  R
H  M  T  M  H  E  I  S  N  T  Y  V  O
E  I  H  I  M  G  Y  R  Y  I  E  I  F
R  A  G  O  C  N  G  E  L  W  A  D  E
```

AGITATED	INSOMNIA	SNORING
ANXIOUS	JETLAG	STRESSED
ASTIR	LETHARGIC	THINKING
DROWSY	LISTLESS	TIRED
EDGY	RED-EYE	WIDE AWAKE
FORTY WINKS	SHUTEYE	WORRIED

"It is one of life's bitterest truths that bedtime so often arrives just when things are really getting interesting."

Lemony Snicket

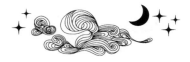

Wedding

```
Y A V O E I I E R A B Z R
A J I D Y H D D F E S M E
P Z I S E S F D T I M O H
L R F I L S R R U G W S P
B E S L E E O P E N W E A
E D K G S T G R O O M T R
S L A S H T N E V A E B G
A P R E N I E E T A T S O
F H D H O N E Y M O O N T
R E C E P T I O N A G J O
N D A R O S A L T A R M H
Y I R S U O D B E B M R P
E J S K T H Y S T A R G Y
I N T A S U C S E S S I K
D N A B S U H A R I E H U
```

AISLE   DRESS   MARRY
ALTAR   FEAST   PAGES
BETROTHED   GROOM   PHOTO-
BRIDE   HONEYMOON   GRAPHER
CARS   HUSBAND   RECEPTION
CHURCH   KISSES   VOWS
                              WIFE

In our dreams—Marriage:

It is likely that a marriage or wedding within
a dream would indicate the need for two
parts of the dreamer to be better connected;
the physical and spiritual for example.

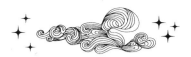

Dream and Sleep Demons of Folklore

```
S D E B B E G A H D L O E
H A K K A T O M E R A W R
A M M U T T A D O R I N A
D E A S I S B E B A P N M
O I D H B A B S I G R D P
W G A S A N H A R V S H O
P F E B T D B L A H I T A
E E E K G F D R A A M L T
O B S H E T Y I M P P I E
P C O A H P T L E M E E S
L T R P N A E B U L S T I
E O G A N T I A N A A O N
M D S S W P A E C R F N E
T R H A S U B U C N I I V
O A M O K O K E T J V S M
```

AMMUTTADORI	KOKOMA	PESANTA
BATIBAT	LIETONIS	PHI AM
HADDIELA	MARE	SHADOW
INCUBUS	MORA	PEOPLE
JINN	MOTAKKA	SHAITAN
KHAPASA	OLD HAG	VARYPNAS
		VRAHNAS

"Evil in general does not sleep, and therefore doesn't see why anyone else should."

Neil Gaiman and Terry Pratchett

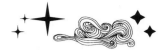

Twinkle, Twinkle, Little Star

```
T W I K Y E N O G S E H T
K N F K U E O A T A R R J
E U S L T S P A R K A R H
E S B I Y I R D H V M I L
P G N I Z A L B E T G R I
T Y T P D U W L E H S E G
W W I H O R L B V A E D H
S G I C O E D R O N N N T
N N N R U P I B K I O S
N I I K A G G A S H W W
E S G A H L Y H O W S E O
T H A H T T E T T U H S R
F O U R T R O E L T T I L
O W P E E P U N K N O W D
D N O M A I D C E K R A D
```

Twinkle, twinkle, little star,
How I wonder what you are!
Up above the world so high,
Like a diamond in the sky.

When the blazing sun is gone,
When he nothing shines upon,
Then you show your little light,
Twinkle, twinkle all the night.

Then the traveller in the dark,
Thanks you for your tiny spark,
He could not see which way to go,
If you did not twinkle so.

In the dark blue sky you keep,
And often through my curtains peep,
For you never shut your eye,
'til the sun is in the sky.

As your bright and tiny spark,
Lights the traveller in the dark,
Though I know not what you are,
Twinkle, twinkle, little star.

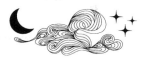

Cell Phone

```
L C A D O P G L O B M E W
A E N T R A S T I K M E F
N J H C A L L E R I D G S
G N F E I S E M T S P A H
I E R E A K N K M G A R B
S T Y R F D A T A I D E Y
G W P G P E S R E H D V B
I O P C P S A E T A R O D
N R N E K U S E T E E C N
S K U I I E P K B E S K A
A M N G M E M O R Y S E T
G S A A L A R M T K B T S
S O G R J O K E Y L O C K
T E U T T G N I M A O R C
I M D I G I T A L E K A S
```

ADDRESS BOOK	GPRS	ROAMING
ALARM	HEADSET	SIGNAL
CALLER ID	KEY LOCK	SKINS
COVERAGE	MEMORY	SMART
DIGITAL	NETWORK	STANDBY
GAMES	PEAK TIME	TOP-UP

Sleep tip—Blue light free zone:

Blue light prevents the secretion of the sleep hormone melatonin. Cut screens out of your bedtime routine and try a puzzle or reading a book instead.

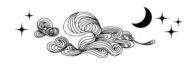

9   Words That Follow "DAY"

BED   LIGHTS
BOOK   ROOM
BREAK   SPRING
CARE   TIME
DREAMER   WORKERS

```
G A T G N I R P S
U S R E K R O W D
A R M L Y N L R D
I I O U K E E N Y
T I Y O E A A B D
D U G B M V E E E
I C O E R A C R B
I O R I G R O W B
K M S T H G I L S
```

10   Bright

AGLOW   LUMINOUS
DAZZLING   RADIANT
GLEAMING   SHINING
GOLDEN   SUNNY
LIGHT   VIVID

```
W O L G A D G S S
G S H I N I N G U
N G U D I V I V O
I U N N E I L G N
M A B I N U Z U I
A I F N A Y Z R M
E T N A I D A R U
L I G H T C D E L
G A O N E D L O G
```

"It was the possibility of darkness that made the day seem so bright."

Stephen King

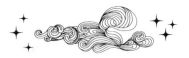

Muscles

```
G N I R T S E Y E B W C S
A B R I C O P S S T A Y P
R S U I N E L P S I D S E
K S U C C P E U D A U P C
E U U A R C S R Y E S E I
S E G T I C A O D R U C B
D L S R C C G I A I I T H
I O T U S E O U S S D O G
O S O L C B R C C O E R L
T O R R M A A L A R P A U
L M S O T L I T N I A L T
E L H A E N B L Y U T I E
D R E N R U P V I S S S U
W S U I Z E P A R T E A S
K S P R O N A T O R T O R
```

BICEPS   PECTORALIS   SCALENUS
CARDIAC   PRONATOR   SOLEUS
DELTOID   PSOAS   SPLENIUS
EYE-STRING   RECTUS   STAPEDIUS
GLUTEUS   RHOMBOIDEUS   TRAPEZIUS
ILIACUS   RISORIUS   TRICEPS

Sleep fact

A hypnic jerk is suddenly jumping awake as you
fall asleep. You may experience a falling sensation,
quickened heart-rate, and sweating. Around 70% of
people experience them at some point in their lives
and they are thought to be completely benign.

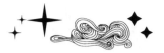

Owls

```
V  I  F  L  G  E  P  B  S  I  C  B  I
S  C  E  L  C  O  P  W  U  O  A  P  G
T  D  E  E  E  T  C  M  Y  R  O  N  T
R  M  O  R  E  P  O  R  K  N  I  T  U
I  E  F  U  M  L  L  I  G  W  W  O  Y
P  Y  G  M  Y  M  N  I  O  I  P  A  L
E  F  L  M  O  G  P  R  T  G  B  H  T
D  A  I  A  N  S  R  H  V  T  M  U  F
O  S  E  R  A  U  W  L  M  L  L  V  C
O  A  A  S  B  Y  O  B  V  E  L  E  O
W  B  C  H  F  U  L  V  O  U  S  N  C
H  F  D  E  T  T  O  P  S  S  W  V  A
V  W  O  H  C  E  E  R  C  S  A  S  H
L  I  T  T  E  A  D  E  T  S  E  R  C
L  N  S  N  O  W  Y  B  D  L  A  B  C
```

BARKING	FULVOUS	SNOWY
BARN	LITTLE	SOOTY
BURROWING	MARSH	SPOTTED
CHACO	MOREPORK	STRIPED
CRESTED	PYGMY	TAWNY
ELF	SCREECH	WOOD

"We love the night and its quiet; and there is no night that we love so well as that on which the moon is coffined in clouds."

Fitz James O'Brien

Education

```
S U I N O I T I U T S U A
C X D E Q O U A E C U N V
I O F O R L D S O O D A I
E S A C O U T U N T C M E
N T E C S S T T H Z V A T
C T K A H R I C H S H S A
E E U G H B E I E I E T U
R E D T O I C T G L N E D
S N O X O X Y H S L O R A
L I L A I R S E Z E O X R
N M Y T E C A O Z Y M R G
G A C K H E S R Q D R E T
K X E O T V T Y A U A U S
N E O D S T A T U T E S O
N L P R O C T O R S T U P
```

COACH   MASTER   STATUTES
DEAN   POSTGRADUATE STUDY
EXAMINEE PROCTOR   TESTS
HIGH SCHOOL SCIENCE   THEORY
LECTURE   SCOUT   TUITION
LOCKER   SEMESTER TUTOR

In our dreams—Exams and tests:

This may indicate a form of self-criticism
and a desire for high achievement.

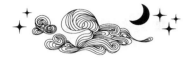

Sleep Diary

Make a record of how you slept this week
to see where you can improve.

Here are some useful facts to record and monitor:

- Time of going to bed
- Time it took to fall asleep
- Number of times you awoke
- Time spent awake
- Total hours of sleep
- Notes and observations

Monday

....
....
....

Tuesday

....
....
....

Wednesday

....
....
....

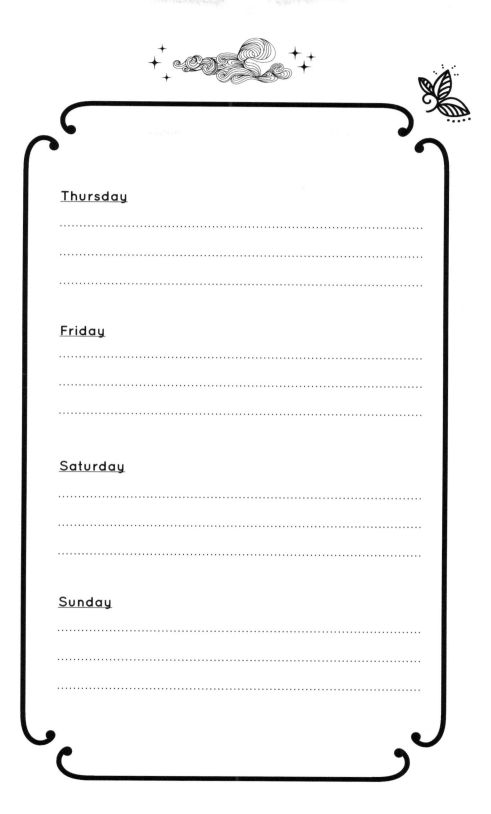

Thursday

....

....

....

Friday

....

....

....

Saturday

....

....

....

Sunday

....

....

....

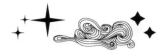

Night-related Deities

```
M L Y O M I L A H S E B E
P O T M D A A B A T A B H
I H R E O Y N H A Y E N F
A E A P C V S U R O H C S
T R U I H I G O L I A N E
S E Y P R E T R M N M I L
K B H A S E U L L N L A E
E U A V R V T S U T U S N
R S L O N D I S Z A O S E
B R Q F A I N T A N H H V
T L A A S O E A P T L O U
F S U T H M H Y H E I A Y
N N M K R M H N N C L F D
V Y F V G I I A S A N E D
R V X E W S I M E T R A L
```

AHRIMAN	EREBUS	NYX
AL-QAUM	HYPNOS	RATRI
ARTEMIS	KHONSU	SELENE
ASTERIA	LUNA	SHALIM
BREKSTA	METZTLI	SOMNUS
CHANDRA	MORPHEUS	YOHAULTICETL

"We are such stuff
As dreams are made on; and our little life
Is rounded with a sleep."

William Shakespeare

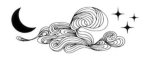

Anatomy

```
C H T H P A S V E G C D B
C U A I P L E E R O K I M
G J J Q O R B S L P S N E
E J A C T G H O T G H W E
S G W E F I N N Y C Y S K
E T B C N P E R I U T O H
H R O S U T E V M S S L N
A P N M C A A O P U S E O
M W E T A I T I D O M G O
U O F Z R C N C R O R E Y
I B O I I E H E D H A C F
L L O V N B L B C M Y P Y
I E T Y E G A O E L C E H
S A G E L I E X T A W A T
O L H S E S E R O P E R D
```

ABDOMEN	GUT	SHIN
ARMS	ILIUM	SOLE
COLON	JAWBONE	SPINE
ELBOW	LEGS	STOMACH
FINGER	PALM	VERTEBRA
FOOT	PORES	VOICE BOX

In our dreams—Teeth falling out:

This may represent going through a transition, perhaps as from childhood to adulthood, or adulthood to old age and may indicate anxiety about growing older.

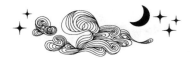

16   # Comediennes

BALL   SAUNDERS
BRAND   SYKES
BURNETT   TOMLIN
DILLER   ULLMAN
RIVERS   WOOD

```
S R E D N U A S T
N I L L D S O T F
D V I L E N E S T
I E H K B N A O I
L R Y A R L M R D
L S L U N L Y O B
E L B H I L O I V
R Y O N G W M C T
L N A M L L U S A
```

17   # Fighting Talk

BOUT   FRAY
BRAWL   HOSTILE
COMBAT   MELEE
DUEL   SKIRMISH
FEUD   STRUGGLE

```
A E L G G U R T S
E M E Y M C Y K O
E A D V O R I B S
L T L M F R B H F
E T B E M R R O E
M A U I U C A M U
T O S O E D W Y D
A H F H B B L E E
T E L I T S O H D
```

"Never go to bed mad. Stay up and fight."

Phyllis Diller

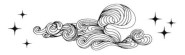

Flying Machines

```
M I C R O L I G H T J K A
P I M A S E L W L U R I P
M Y R T Y I M T M E R N I
I E S A D T S P T S C T T
L E T E G H J P H R P U C
B D R S U E O I P E R P H
T M E T T H P C H B U S I
L E T N T Z E P P E L I N
I L K I O A U T O G I R O
E J N C P R N S E P A O O
L R E R O H D B A U N A K
O H E U T R I P L A N E B
N O O L L A B B L U M P M
T F A R C E C A P S S E E
P A I R K W A H K C A L B
```

AIRSHIP	DRONE	ROCKET
AUTOGIRO	GLIDER	SHUTTLE
BALLOON	JUMP JET	SPACECRAFT
BLACK HAWK	MICROLIGHT	SPUTNIK
BLIMP	MIRAGE	TRIPLANE
CHINOOK	ORNITHOPTER	ZEPPELIN

In our dreams—Flying:

This may signal that we are releasing ourselves of
our inhibitions and allowing ourselves to be free.

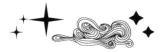

```
T  J  F  L  A  D  N  A  G  S  P  S  E
I  A  L  E  N  E  R  H  A  H  N  A  A
B  O  E  O  W  Y  N  B  T  I  E  A  R
B  V  R  R  Z  I  G  Y  G  R  S  L  E
O  E  A  C  H  S  Z  G  Y  E  E  L  G
H  A  Y  B  S  W  A  A  R  I  E  D  R
C  O  D  E  S  B  L  L  R  V  J  U  R
A  D  C  B  O  S  E  D  E  D  B  N  G
R  U  J  B  E  G  A  N  M  R  R  M  N
I  B  L  Y  U  L  T  N  E  O  U  A  I
S  I  S  A  A  Y  L  T  G  L  R  I  L
B  E  T  G  O  P  T  A  L  O  Q  R  M
K  Y  Q  N  T  U  R  O  H  V  D  O  A
A  C  E  E  B  A  G  A  G  L  Y  M  G
L  E  D  O  O  I  N  S  I  M  B  E  R
```

ARAGORN	EOWYN	MERRY
ARWEN	GALADRIEL	MORIA
BILBO BAGGINS	GAMLING	ORCS
BUTTERBUR	GANDALF	ROHAN
ELEVENTY-ONE	GOLLUM	SHIRE
ELF	HOBBIT	WIZARD

"Now not day only shall be beloved,
but night too shall be beautiful and
blessed and all its fear pass away!"

J.R.R. Tolkien

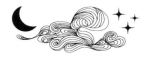

20   Bath Time

CALM   SOAK
RELAX   SOAP
ROBE   TOWEL
SHAMPOO   UNWIND
SLIPPERS   WASH

```
H P A O S E S B U
C A L M X D R U S
U S W A S H N S L
A O L O E W H V I
E E A B I A L P P
R K O N M S E S P
V R D P N B W F E
O E O E X A O V R
D O E P D D T C S
```

21   Words From the Letters in "PATTERNS"

ASTER   PATENT
EARNS   PEARS
NAPE   RASP
NEAR   TRANSEPT
PARENTS   TREAT

```
T N A R N T E T R
S T E E A P E N E
T A A P P E A E R
N R R T E S R T T
E R S N T N E A S
R A S E R A E P R
A S R A T R T E A
P A S N T T N R E
T P E P S T P T P
```

Sleep tip—Keep sleep regular:

A regular sleep pattern, getting up at the same time (even at the weekend!), and avoiding napping where possible can all aid in a better sleep pattern.

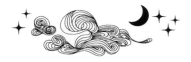

Winning

```
D N O I T C A F S I T A S
R N Y F A V I H A V E L A
A S E H I M P S E D O R E
W T P D E A U H D M A F A
A R A R Y C U G R T A M I
K E S A C H N O Y N C G L
M B L E U I S I B A B U E
A E S Y A E P E A R E A P
R S L C T V A A E G Y T M
A P C T E E L G S H U E M
T U E K G M D M P S S S H
H M N A O E O O X E T B A
O P E W U N R M E D A L S
N S A N E T Y E Z I R P G
S W E Y P T E R B I L I T
```

ACHIEVEMENT	GRANT	RELAY
AWARD	MARATHON	ROSETTE
CUP	MEDALS	SATISFACTION
EDGE	MONEY	STAR
GAIN	PASS	SUCCESS
GAME	PRIZE	TROPHY

"One good night's sleep can help you realize that you shouldn't break up with someone, or you are being too hard on your friend, or you actually will win the race or the game or get the job. Sleep helps you win at life."

Amy Poehler

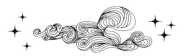

"NIGHT" Words

```
K O C L A E R N I E T E S
R W R L A F D F O L L R F
O I A V O I J J G I U H B
W N W Y F L E A G J S B E
E G L R J W H H N E P I J
C R E D A G T E G E Y C V
Q L R Y O J B Y Y L E N W
L I O W E O E O H B C I A
B B N T J E L W R A B Y T
K A I P H B L R E L W Y C
N A V R L E C S E W L K H
M A R E I K S P A C B J M
O G G D J E R L W E A R A
W B L I N D N E S S A S N
L A V R L U N A R E R E D
```

BELL	GOWN	OWL
BIRD	HAWK	RIDER
BLINDNESS	JAR	VISION
CAP	LIFE	WATCHMAN
CLOTHES	LIGHT	WEAR
CRAWLER	MARE	WORK

Sleep fact

In the past it was common to get up for a few hours in the middle of the night. This time was used to read, engage in activities, or spend time with others.

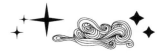

24   Words From the Letters in "GOODNIGHT"

DHOTI   GOTH

DIG   HOOD

GIN   HOOTING

GOING   NIGHT

GONG   ONTO

```
O G O N N H G I H
G G H I O I G I G
N G O H N D G G O
I I N H O O I H I
O G T I I O O O T
G D G G T I D D O
H N H N D O I D H
I G O T H G O H D
T G T G T T T H N
```

25   Night-time Noises

BABIES   DOGS

BUMPS   FOXES

CARS   OWLS

CATS   PLANES

CRICKETS   TRAINS

```
L S L U S H D P N
C R P L V O S M S
A A W G G P E N H
E O R S D L I D S
S C V S U A B Y P
E U A U R N A N M
X Y I T V E B C U
O I U P S S G S B
F S T E K C I R C
```

"Goodnight stars, goodnight air,
goodnight noises everywhere."

Margaret Wise Brown

Scottish Lochs

```
L A Y G N O F R U A B E R
R E A E V E R N I R R Y C
N A V E R O K O C D E A M
U E B O I R K S M T D H L
L E S C F Y K C O D E O P
G E G S B S Q T A U Q S N
H M I E N I A G G N I A K
W A I G G I Y A H V Y H E
N E S A G E I Q E R E G S
A E R D L D U N A P O O L
M O V L H Y I O B L A P M
E O A H Z R H T U R C T E
O V R R T E E L A S O N R
A T R A N U S A N E R O R
H J K C R A R W B L O O M
```

BROOM   MORAR   RYAN
GAINEIMH   NAVER   SUNART
GYNACK   NESS   TOTAIG
KATRINE   NEVIS   UNAPOOL
LEVEN   RIDDON   VALLEY
MHEUGAIDH   RUTHVEN   WALTON

In our dreams—Drowning:
This may indicate we are in danger of being emotionally overwhelmed and perhaps afraid of being honest with our emotions.

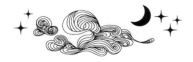

```
N T H J M E L L I V L E M
I R C H A N D L E R V V F
A F V E M M H Y N Y U G I
W F F Y I C E E S D G L M
T P P L S H C S L T L N O
P S L D Y O D A B L A Y R
T E C L F G R P R M E E R
R V O N N E G U T T K R I
H T G B G H O I P L H M S
I F R Z E R H C A D V Y O
S A T U R W Y W O Y I O N
D I C K I N S O N N G K I
F E S C A U O R E K N L E
Y G K C E B N I E T S O U
R R E N K L U A F A V O R
```

CHANDLER	KEROUAC	STEINBECK
DICKINSON	MCCARTHY	TWAIN
FAULKNER	MELVILLE	UPDIKE
FITZGERALD	MILLER	VONNEGUT
HELLER	MORRISON	WALKER
JAMES	O'CONNOR	WHITMAN

"It is a common experience that a problem difficult at night is resolved in the morning after the committee of sleep has worked on it."

John Steinbeck

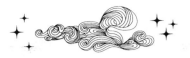

Getting Active

```
S O G W P W H A O R O G I
Y W N R L I G B T J N L H
R U I M U O L A W I U G S
T B B M Y N I A W W R D E
N A M C M R N O T U P J O
U R I Y E I R I G E U I U
O R L C N R N B N J S V M
C E C L H E Y G I G L E B
S O R I G I W T N U A C H
S U I N V R S P G B I N O
O W A G W U E R M D C A I
R I T T L A D U M R F D N
C F S F L S Z D H V Y Y G
K I C K B O X I N G Y O R
A R C A P A R I E O P A C
```

BARRE

CAPOEIRA

CROSS-
   COUNTRY

CYCLING

DANCE

JUDO

JUJITSU

KICKBOXING

PILATES

ROWING

RUGBY

RUNNING

SOCCER

STAIR CLIMBING

SWIMMING

TAI CHI

YOGA

ZUMBA

Sleep tip—Get active:

Exercise in the daytime can aid in better sleep,
avoid anything too vigorous right before
sleep but walking or yoga may help.

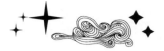

Cats' Names

```
M E A H T N A M A S Y A L
K I B A B E C N C L E Y E
M I S S Y I S W U L D V R
U K T Y I K A L O L E D M
N K U T T I C K T Y Y O A
T D A R Y K H D Q S B T R
R H E R A S L L S D M B M
I R L E S E E A S A I I A
N Y D E I R S A C I S N L
I B V F I M C H V S I E A
S E R R W K E O U Y M A D
H A R N C S O E N T B R E
G R E S T T R O A A A M B
S R G E S U O I C E R P C
I H R U M A E R A S Z O E
```

ABBY	GARFIELD	MISSY
BEAR	KIKI	PRECIOUS
CHESTER	KITTY	SAMANTHA
CLEO	LOLA	SASSY
COOKIE	LUNA	SIMBA
DAISY	MARMALADE	ZOE

Sleep fact

Humans spend, on average, 1/3 of their lives asleep
but cats sleep for a whopping 2/3 of theirs!

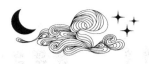

30   Words From the Letters in "SUNRISE"

REINS   SIREN
RINSE   SUNS
RISEN   URN
RUIN   URSINE
SINUS   USER

```
R R I U N R N S E
S N N R R E I N S
U I U S E I I U N
S U E U R R N I I
U R U N N U E R R
S S U I I S S R E
E U N S U S I I U
R U E N S I R E N
N I S E S S N U R
```

31   Beauty

ALLURE   GRACE
APPEAL   LOVELY
BEAUTY   PLEASANT
CHARM   PRETTY
ELEGANCE   STYLISH

```
E L E G A N C E B
L R O C A Y H Y P
A R U G A S F T L
E N E L I R C U O
P U I L L H G A V
P V Y U A A T E E
A T I R E S O B L
S Y M P R E T T Y
T N A S A E L P A
```

"There is no sunrise so beautiful that
it is worth waking me up to see it."

Mindy Kaling

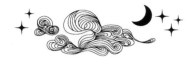

```
S  P  H  C  T  A  W  T  E  K  C  O  P
R  E  D  Q  U  E  E  N  D  N  O  B  K
I  P  L  U  A  S  K  R  K  A  O  R  E
D  P  N  E  S  R  I  K  A  V  K  I  R
D  E  B  E  P  N  I  D  R  E  A  M  A
L  R  V  Z  K  E  R  E  V  O  S  N  H
E  E  D  M  F  A  T  A  Y  F  U  G  H
S  C  E  U  E  T  F  E  R  H  R  I  C
E  I  D  F  A  M  E  H  Y  E  L  C  R
H  L  N  H  C  E  A  R  R  A  A  E  A
J  A  D  J  F  N  O  O  D  R  W  M  M
P  A  K  O  I  L  S  L  S  T  T  S  O
M  G  B  D  A  E  O  I  R  S  R  D  U
A  E  V  E  S  S  O  R  S  T  O  E  O
R  A  E  S  U  O  M  R  O  D  K  C  U
```

ALICE	DRINK ME	PEPPER
COOK	EAT ME	POCKET WATCH
DINAH	KNAVE OF	RED QUEEN
DODO	HEARTS	RIDDLES
DORMOUSE	LORY	ROSES
DREAM	MAD HATTER	WALRUS
	MARCH HARE	

In our dreams—Falling:

This may indicate a lack of confidence in ourselves
or that we feel a lack of security in our lives.

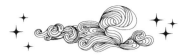

Science Fiction TV

```
L M E P A C S R A F S G A
E H E F R A W D D E R V N
L P G S O O B S L G P N D
L D D A N H S I T Y R M R
I D M O O A F W R I H V O
V E O W O X P A E M B S M
R Y Y C E W U X U L L S E
O Y L H T T H U E I L T D
E F T F C O N C D E I A A
H F R N E I R E R M H R H
T U A I T R R W E O D T Y
Y S M N N S I L H V T R O
M C O A O G E F O O S E S
G C B B N S E E U R E K A
O L R D S S N D F I V W W
```

ANDROMEDA	FRINGE	STAR TREK
CONTINUUM	HUMANS	THE EXPANSE
DOCTOR WHO	RED DWARF	THE ORVILLE
EUREKA	ROSWELL	THE X FILES
FARSCAPE	SANCTUARY	TIMELESS
FIREFLY	SLIDERS	TORCHWOOD

"He felt that his whole life was some kind of dream and he sometimes wondered whose it was and whether they were enjoying it."

Douglas Adams

Monsters

```
N D B O G E Y M A N I D U
D A S H S U H G C I N E O
E E F G L E G S H E L O B
A G S D R E L A T A R A R
N S G T D E A W L R E I I
Y B U O R I T E Y A N F E
F L R D D O F T O P N Y Z
M A H N E Z Y Y I S V N G
R C S X K M I E M R M N A
D K V O Y E L L R A I X P
S A R T L S H R L H C M J
M N Y A Y T D Y T A A R D
A N K S K O L E D H S A A
U I O T K E H U C R E F G
G S Y F R T N A P I A K E
```

AGGEDOR	GODZILLA	MEDUSA
BLACK ANNIS	GRETTIR	SHELOB
BOGEYMAN	GUGALANNA	SLEIPNIR
CHAMP	HYDRA	SMAUG
DESTROYER	KRAKEN	THE THING
FASOLT	MACRA	YETI

In our dreams—Monsters:

This is likely related to something we have allowed to become larger than life, allowing it to appear as a creature. It may indicate a negative relationship with our own emotions.

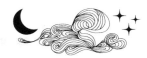

Baseball Hall of Famers

```
A F E U O U L V M D H E B
R F F I E S F A C Y X I T
R R S N I L L O C X F O O
E I W O V A C M O A I J R
B S N S R U S F I A T A E
N C F N P G T G E G M L R
O H H H P H O M G Y P L R
F R T O L T A O C O M E E
I U K J R E S F S G B W U
R H O E N R D I W B R G G
S Y T D I D C H M Y D A D
J E N N I N G S M M V B W
J H H M A T H E W S O N T
F Y L S D U D C W T C N A
S I R R A H I T O Y H M S
```

BAGWELL   GUERRERO   MATHEWSON
BERRA   HARRIS   MCGRAW
BOGGS   JENNINGS   NIEKRO
COLLINS   JETER   RUTH
FOXX   JOHNSON   SIMMONS
FRISCH   LAJOIE   SLAUGHTER

"I usually take a two-hour
nap from one to four."

Yogi Berra

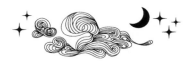

Sleep Inhibiting Food and Drinks

```
H  S  I  D  A  R  W  Y  T  M  R  R  E
B  D  U  D  W  H  L  D  T  M  T  T  P
V  R  C  G  B  E  A  N  S  N  A  O  A
G  C  O  I  A  V  H  A  H  L  D  L  O
N  E  F  C  L  R  O  C  O  H  C  C  P
S  Y  F  R  C  W  R  C  W  O  A  B  H
N  T  E  D  C  O  O  D  H  H  H  M  M
A  C  E  O  S  H  L  O  I  U  E  L  O
T  N  V  A  C  F  L  I  T  M  L  Y  T
S  O  C  K  K  C  U  B  E  D  L  N  A
A  C  R  E  C  A  E  D  B  D  M  B  M
P  A  A  D  Y  D  V  L  R  H  N  R  O
D  B  A  K  B  O  N  L  E  H  R  I  T
S  Y  U  F  E  S  D  A  A  R  A  E  E
L  L  O  L  F  T  F  N  D  V  Y  D  U
```

ALCOHOL
BACON
BEANS
BRIE
BROCCOLI
CAKE

CANDY
CELERY
COFFEE
DARK
  CHOCOLATE
HAM
PASTA

RADISH
SODA
STEAK
SUGAR
TOMATO
WHITE BREAD

Sleep tip—Don't eat before bed:

Eating a large meal shortly before going to bed
has been shown to suppress the secretion of
melatonin, so try to eat earlier in the evening.

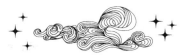

Magical

```
E L X E O M L U G C G L F
L A R U T A N N U N Y A A
D E X C T C I S I R L E N
R D R E A M Y H A J D R C
I N G N D V C D S N R N I
E E N N W T N A O E A U F
W Y K N I E R F R N Z R U
C B K W G F V T C C I G L
E I R E E S L U E H W N I
S K L S G R A E R A I I S
H C T I R D L E O N I M H
F B R A T L M T U T T R E
N E H G A H N E S I O A S
E T Y L A N E M O N E H P
F Y L T S O H G A G L C E
```

CHARMING	FANCIFUL	UNCANNY
DREAMY	FEY	UNNATURAL
EERIE	GHOSTLY	UNREAL
ELDRITCH	LEGENDARY	WEIRD
ELFIN	PHENOMENAL	WITCHING
ENCHANTING	SORCEROUS	WIZARDLY

"The night is darkening round me,
The wild winds coldly blow;
But a tyrant spell has bound me
And I cannot, cannot go."

Emily Brontë

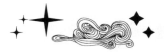

Feeling Refreshed

Make a list of all of the things, people, and activities
that make you feel peaceful and refreshed. Once you've
made your list make a conscious effort to include more
of these things in your life.

For example, do you always feel reinvigorated
after going for a run? Is there a particular friend
who helps to boost your emotional well-being? Or
do you feel better from simply finding time to curl
up with a good book?

1. ....

2. ....

3. ....

4. ....

5. ....

6. ....

7. ....

8. ....

9. ....

10. ....

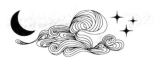

Animals with Unusual Sleeping Habits

```
W F O S E H C I R T S O I
S A I A W T N R V U P N N
R C L C H F R C S R A E B
E G O R T O D S E Y V F D
T S S O U B I M F T N E V
T H K N S S E L F D S L S
O A O Y A E E Y A E C E A
A R A H R M L S R N S P R
E K L K P B U T I Y E H B
S S A B N H S H G S S A E
F T S N A N U W I L R N Z
S R R E A I M L F O O T Y
I L O I S K C U D T H S V
E E L G W D O L P H I N S
F S T F S D T U I S A M I
```

BEARS	GIRAFFES	OSTRICHES
DESERT SNAILS	HORSES	SEA OTTERS
DOLPHINS	HUMANS	SHARKS
DUCKS	KOALAS	SLOTHS
ELEPHANTS	MEERKATS	WALRUSES
FROGS	ORCAS	ZEBRAS

Sleep fact

Humans are the only mammals that are
known to willingly delay sleep.

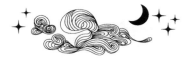

Fictional Sleuths

```
Y R E E E N T H M D A N E
A S P L V Y E C A L X U T
S E C Y M K R Z G I R M O
T E V O P U G Y N E R S R
H O R F L D I N U D C P I
U S H D U U A V M U H E O
E L V T A M M O N K I N P
N E R O G Y B B O B N C E
S L S W E S N N O F V E L
S E N N A M A M E W E R U
O G G M M L I N D O D S C
Y A N N A H D R A H C I R
C Y K E E R C I C H G O E
W K F K A I H I A P P U H
N O S R E D N N B L E T H
```

BOBBY GOREN

CAGNEY

CHAN

COLUMBO

CREEK

FOYLE

HERCULE
   POIROT

LACEY

LAIDLAW

MAGNUM

MAIGRET

MANNIX

MONK

MORSE

RICHARD
   HANNAY

SGT HO

SPENCER

ZEN

In our dreams—Murder:

This may indicate trying to control a part of our nature we do not trust. If we are trying to murder someone we should consider what that person represents to understand the hostility of our feelings.

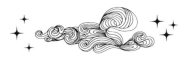

Capital Cities of Europe

```
H A S I H B A L E S A R S
M B E T A B E E O S D N R
W F E I H O S R W N E N G
A E F R V E L C G H D B I
R O J Z N T A I T A L O D
S K O P J E H A S E Z M N
A C A M T C R I Y B V T E
W N E U G A R P E A O J G
K I D A S A L R D U A N A
S L R U P B U U T A I P H
N B A R D U Z H B S S A N
I U H E L S I N K I O S E
M D B O N N I S N G C E P
O M G R U V E D Y B I R O
S U I N L I V I E N N A C
```

ATHENS	LONDON	SOFIA
BERNE	MINSK	VADUZ
COPENHAGEN	NICOSIA	VIENNA
DUBLIN	PARIS	VILNIUS
HELSINKI	PRAGUE	WARSAW
LISBON	SKOPJE	ZAGREB

"I cannot walk through the suburbs in the solitude of the night without thinking that the night pleases us because it suppresses idle details, just as our memory does."

Jorge Luis Borges

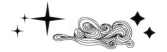

Booker Prize Winners

```
R W L U E R W M F Y I Y O
U L E T N A M C A A G D G
S T S V S S O R W D W M N
H I A G A E W H O I I A U
D S U M T R D O T E G G O
I V U Z G O I S R A N C A
E S E Y O N N S N T E L C
Y E H W O R I A T J H C F
T W T I U H L D T O S R N
T A A B G F M A L W E A D
A N R O R U A E I O W T F
E L Y O D D R F O E G S F
B E T C N B T O C M O S R
R L F O W A E M C W U P A
S E P E C T L U A P I A N
```

ADIGA   EVARISTO   MCEWAN
ATWOOD   FLANAGAN   NAIPAUL
BEATTY   GOLDING   ONDAATJE
BURNS   ISHIGURO   RUSHDIE
COETZEE   MANTEL   SWIFT
DOYLE   MARTEL   UNSWORTH

"You're always in a rush, or else
you're too exhausted to have a proper
conversation. Soon enough, the long
hours, the travelling, the broken sleep
have all crept into your being and become
part of you, so everyone can see it."

Kazuo Ishiguro

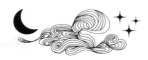

42   Words From the Letters in "PURSUED"

DRUPES	SPED
DUPE	SPUR
PRUDES	SUED
PURE	SUPER
PURSED	USURPED

```
D R S E P U R D U
R U D S R U E R D
U R E R E U D E U
P E P U D E P U R
U R R E E S D R R
R S U S U U U E R
S S S D P S P D D
E R U S E U U P R
D R S S S S R P U
```

43   Escape

ABSCOND	FLEE
BOLT	FLIGHT
BREAKOUT	FREEDOM
DEPART	LEAVE
ESCAPE	VANISH

```
U T M H S I N A V
T U Y O H V T A E
F O A Y D D S P H
R K L B E E A I E
B A E P S C E G Y
O E A I S C O R E
L R V E H O O E F
T B E P I O L N E
T H G I L F G E D
```

In our dreams—Being chased:
We may be trying to escape responsibility, a fear of failure, or other emotions we feel we cannot cope with.

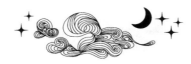

44   Words From the Letters in "SLEEPING"

ELSE	PEELING
GEL	PENS
GENIE	PIGS
GIN	PINE
GLENS	SPLEEN

```
S  E  P  L  L  E  G  L  S
G  I  E  I  S  N  L  S  G
E  S  S  E  I  N  I  L  E
N  P  N  L  E  N  L  I  E
I  L  E  E  I  E  P  P  S
E  E  L  L  P  E  G  G  L
P  P  G  I  P  L  I  G  E
L  I  N  E  I  P  G  I  E
S  E  L  I  G  S  G  N  S
```

45   Love

ADORE	FRIEND
AFFECTION	LIKE
CHERISH	PRIZE
ESTEEM	REGARD
FAMILY	REVERE

```
E  H  S  I  R  E  H  C  E
M  M  Y  L  I  M  A  F  M
F  R  I  E  N  D  V  E  P
N  D  E  R  E  V  E  R  S
A  F  F  E  C  T  I  O  N
L  D  H  H  S  Z  H  N  I
D  I  O  E  E  U  C  A  O
B  A  K  R  E  G  A  R  D
A  U  A  E  E  Y  C  C  V
```

> "I love sleep so much. That's the one thing I won't sacrifice. I really cannot."
>
> *Bozoma Saint John*

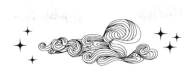

Sleep Inducing Foods and Drinks

```
S E R S E G N A R O S E R
E R A Y E K R U T G A G P
H S I F R L H A P S N P S
A Y S O T F E E A E A E E
S V I U H R A T G P N L O
T U N A O T P E T R A H T
U V S H A O N L L U B O A
N Y S P P L S I S N C N T
L R B C S G M M R E R E O
A A O D G A U O N S S Y P
W R E E E L E M N A E U T
N E C M P C C A N D A I E
S F Y P T Y O H I P S V E
C G A B D A C C I C G U W
E C I R N W O R B V Y W S
```

ALMONDS	HONEY	PRUNES
BANANAS	LETTUCE	RAISINS
BROWN RICE	OATMEAL	SEEDS
CHAMOMILE TEA	ORANGES	SWEET
EGGS	PLUMS	POTATOES
FISH	POPCORN	TURKEY
		WALNUTS

Sleep tip—Cut out caffeine:

Try to avoid or cutdown on caffeine and alcohol
as they not only make it harder to fall asleep, but
also prevent deep restful sleep from occurring.

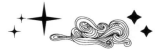

Romanticism

```
G H A V E O Y E H C I N B
I A V D R U N E C F N U S
G V U G N O V A L I S Y N
O P E T Y M G N T L D P R
G B U T I O L A E N E C U
U Y R S E E R E R G E H B
H A W T H O R N E R H R S
O S H E S K O K A E E R B
B E T Y B D I A C B U T N
S W W A C N B N A E L Y T
A C O L E R I D G E I H P
M T O V E K A L B U A T E
U M H T I D R A P O E L Y
D I T T T S N E S A F O G
L Y A D U H L A P S D E P
```

BLAKE	GAUTIER	NOVALIS
BRENTANO	GOETHE	POE
BURNS	HAWTHORNE	PUSHKIN
COLERIDGE	HUGO	SCOTT
DUMAS	KEATS	SHELLEY
GARRETT	LEOPARDI	TIECK

"Oh sleep! it is a gentle thing, Beloved from pole to pole."

Samuel Taylor Coleridge

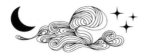

Famous Insomniacs

```
H M S B W L L A R T T A C
A G C D P Y T P A R X L T
L C O I L R A S S O U D C
I H U G M E T B U Y M I T
N G R A N T I W F O P S T
C B D E U A C F A A R S O
O D N G B S V E L I F P A
L K A F K A F A M W N E P
N G L A V B H Y O L E L P
A X R D E N G E N E D B L
B R A J I H D N R M Y Y E
O A G U O V M O O Y E L G
K M K B L N Y O E R V W A
O W H N P M G L A L N C T
V P P A R N E C N A C D E
```

ALDISS	GARLAND	MONROE
APPLEGATE	GRANT	NABOKOV
CAREY	JONG	PALAHNIUK
CATTRALL	KAFKA	PROUST
CLOONEY	LINCOLN	TWAIN
FIELDS	MARX	VAN GOGH

Sleep fact

Insomnia means you regularly experience disrupted
sleeping—this can usually be improved with a change
in habits such as exercise, diet, or dealing with stress
but if this doesn't work you should consult a doctor.

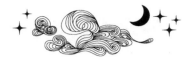

The Moon

```
A P C A N T R U M E M F P
C N O O M F L A H W P H N
V T M H L P S S N Y R O Y
D O G G T Y W E A U O W S
D A R K S I D E S M L C U
G N I X A W D E W A R E P
M M W O T S M E S E H S E
R R W I B W N O S V N P R
E A B C E B A C O G Y I M
V R W R S A E N N N B L O
O Y Y A Y N D I I M S C O
R U F T T A D F G N T E N
S E T E V N M A M Y G E T
E Y F R A V G I B B O U S
E T I L L E T A S T E T D
```

CRATER	LANDING	ROVER
CRESCENT	LUNAR	SATELLITE
DARK SIDE	MOONSET	SUPERMOON
ECLIPSE	NEW MOON	TIDES
GIBBOUS	ORBIT	WANING
HALF MOON	PHASES	WAXING

"There is something haunting in the light of the moon; it has all the dispassionateness of a disembodied soul, and something of its inconceivable mystery."

Joseph Conrad

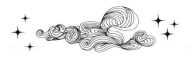

Alone

```
S B U G Z K E R E M O T E
E X J O N O N E S O W N A
P L E H T U O H T I W E C
A X D E D N A R T S R F I
R A H W C Z E E U E H V L
A B G H C J K C C E I O I
T R Z D E S O L A T E U E
E F P C C U G J Y F V Q
V D T L S S Y X J O U Y U
D E S S I V O X R E L E N
D R U V I N P S Z E T T A
N I E Q L N A V N T R S I
B T I Y I K G O X A N O D
S E V X E N L L P V Y L E
V R U N T Z U A E K D O D
```

APART   QUIET   SINGLE
DESOLATE   RECLUSIVE   SOLO
FORSAKEN   REJECTED   STRANDED
LONELY   REMOTE   UNAIDED
ON ONE'S OWN   RETIRED   UNIQUE
ONLY   SEPARATE   WITHOUT HELP

In our dreams—Being Alone:

This can be positive or negative depending on
how we feel in the dream. If negative it may
indicate loneliness or isolation. If positive it
may indicate a need for independence.

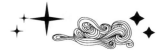

51   Discover

DIG UP	NOTICE
DISCOVER	OBSERVE
FIND	SEEK
INVENT	SPOT
LEARN	UNEARTH

```
V E T A S E H O D
T O P S O L I I L
D N I F E E S P O
I N O A U C E U B
N F R T O F E G S
V N O V I H K I E
E A E B T C L D R
N R N E L Y E C V
T U N E A R T H E
```

52   Great Minds

BELL	NEWTON
CURIE	PLANCK
EDISON	PLATO
FORD	TESLA
KEPLER	WATT

```
O L E G A R T P H
T N E U S L H F P
A H O V T N S L H
L K V S E F A E T
P U E W I N O T T
A U T P C D A R M
S O M K L W E P D
N C U R I E D M C
L L E B H A R L U
```

"Discover the great ideas that lie inside you by discovering the power of sleep."

Arianna Huffington

Things That Help Us Relax

```
G N I R E T T U L C E D N
R S F E A S R N E I I E Y
U O E B U P E A D S F L S
F S I L R R T U U U D A N
P Y P E Z H H B T M R V E
T A I F E Z G E I A A Y Y
T K I O R E U R L N W L S
I G M N U C A P O I I S D
P L A N T S L O S M N R N
I G S P A I U A A A G E E
Y A S U N E N F M L D A I
S M A P Y E O G Y S I D R
V E G N I K O O C Y S I F
C S E A Y G G I S H P N U
E V S E A A I E I Y E G R
```

ANIMALS	GAMES	PLANTS
COOKING	LAUGHTER	PUZZLES
DECLUTTERING	MASSAGE	READING
DRAWING	MUSIC	REIKI
FAMILY	NATURE	SOLITUDE
FRIENDS	PAINTING	YOGA

Sleep tip—A relaxing routine:

Come up with, and stick to a bedtime routine that
you find relaxing, this may involve meditation,
an activity, or a peaceful beauty treatment.

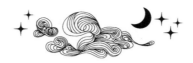

Nursery Rhymes and Stories

```
J A R E P I P D E I P T M
R A Y C S E T C R D R A L
R F R O L W I J W O L R E
D E E N G L E N L R E P S
A L D R A L A L B E T S N
B H R H C T I W A M E K A
N E I N E G H E F V R C H
I N D P J N H P L Y G A S
S A I Y U T H E L B I J H
R E N D A M E S O O R R U
V W G N D I P P A B D E D
A V H E D A E K X I R U D
M V O W F E L G I A N T R
P V O A P W D A L N L P L
E U D S E R N B A D E R G
```

ALADDIN	GRETEL	RED RIDING
ALICE	HANSEL	HOOD
BO PEEP	JACK SPRAT	RUDOLPH
ELVES	PIED PIPER	SINBAD
GENIE	PUMPKIN	TROLL
GIANT	RED HEN	WENDY
		WITCH

"That's the advantage of insomnia.
People who go to bed early always
complain that the night is too short, but
for those of us who stay up all night,
it can feel as long as a lifetime."

Banana Yoshimoto

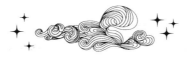

NASA Missions

```
Y U Y B R E G A Y O V M R
O R A U A R O G C Y G E O
R O R E R L R S R A E H A
I A L W I C Y U N N S R D
G P N L S S C K O F D P H
I M Y G O R A I S N H C M
N A T O E P P N A O H R R
S G U M A R A H U S T U E
H E O D I S C O V E R Y Z
U L C S T A R D U S T E T
B L S V U F M O U V M U I
B A S S S I S E N E G F P
L N R G E M I N I U Y I S
E R A G N I K I V P J F R
W A M M U T Y I E D A F D
```

APOLLO	JUNO	RANGER
CHANDRA	MAGELLAN	SKYLAB
DISCOVERY	MARS SCOUT	SPITZER
GEMINI	MERCURY	STARDUST
GENESIS	ORIGINS	VIKING
HUBBLE	PIONEER ·	VOYAGER

Sleep fact

According to NASA the optimum length
of time for a nap is 26 minutes.

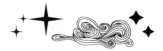

Cradle Song
William Blake

```
D E S I R E S W H E R E L
D T S U O B R I G H T A T
E R A O M A S M I L E S S
L A E I R B E A U T Y W E
T C L A B R E A S T E I T
T E F A M R O M A E Y L F
I H T O D I O W T E P E O
L G T I S R N Z S L R S S
S C U N N I N G E U E R Y
Y A F I G F C E R F T H P
O B N H E H A H K D T K E
J G T C W F E N E A Y A E
H E A R T E E G T E W E L
A F Y B C R E E P R K R S
T E R C E S S P L D Y B A
```

Sleep, sleep, beauty bright,

Dreaming in the joys of night;

Sleep, sleep; in thy sleep,

Little sorrows sit and weep.

Sweet babe, in thy face,

Soft desires I can trace,

Secret joys and secret smiles,

Little pretty infant wiles.

As thy softest limbs I feel,

Smiles as of the morning steal,

O'er thy cheek, and o'er thy breast,

Where thy little heart doth rest.

O the cunning wiles that creep,

In thy little heart asleep!

When thy little heart doth wake,

Then the dreadful night shall break.

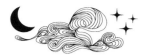

Roald Dahl Characters

```
S A M E E M R O W W O L G
E O P C M S I G G O B C L
T I N H O R T E N S I A R
H U M A S M F H R E F O E
B I D R U O A O E S A N D
Y E U L E N P T X B O E I
N Y E I Y T T H I R F F P
N N A E B P H S I L R G S
A V R B I E P E P E D C S
D O C U S N M O T I V A S
G M S C N A R G H W K O I
T E C K A L F I E R I E M
L A V E N D E R E P M T R
H A W T A B N O R M E V S
M A K N O W Y L L I W U F
```

ALFIE	DANNY	MR FOX
AUNT SPIKER	GLOW-WORM	MR HOPPY
BEAN	HORTENSIA	SOPHIE
BOGGIS	LAVENDER	THE BFG
BUNCE	MATILDA	THE TWITS
CHARLIE BUCKET	MISS SPIDER	WILLY WONKA

"'Dreams is very mystical things,' the BFG said. 'Human beans is not understanding them at all. Not even their brainiest professors is understanding them...'"

Roald Dahl

Warm Words

```
K F D E H S U L F G E V P
I Q L T M C A G L L J U G
A T B A S O B G E N I A L
O V E N C L U C K F T U F
S F U S A I T E I Y K Y X
U G I N U R P C F E N E I
S T K R I N Y O W K R T M
G E L C E R S A R O Q A O
T N I Y E S R H D T C R T
S T I M Z M I C I A N E S
Y K M T G D O D H N P P U
H U E I A V E C E I E M N
S Z E O E E X H D F R E N
L D E R R D H S N B N T Y
E K R B A L M Y L R N K F
```

BALMY	FLUSHED	SUMMERY
BLANKET	GENIAL	SUNNY
COAL	HEATING	SUNSHINE
COVER	LUKEWARM	TEMPERATE
ELECTRICITY	OVEN	TEPID
FIRESIDE	SNUG	TROPICAL

"Don't fight with your pillow,
but lay down your head
And kick every worriment out of the bed."

Edmund Vance Cooke

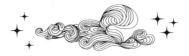

Quiet Words

```
O F I N A U D I B L E G P
O H Y D E I W A D E A E E
S E C L U D E D C B D N A
S F E I L D A F P A S T C
M I V L I G I E R E M L E
H R L C U D H L D R N E F
S F A E Q D E T U M I G U
A L R E N R G H T E A B L
P R I Y A C E U S G R L E
D I G R R S E P G U I R N
A I P W T U N E S T H M E
M L A C S I D N S I G E R
P I R O M E Y V O U H F E
E P F V E T A D E S P W S
N T F L E S A L V A R L I
```

CALM	INAUDIBLE	SERENE
DAMPEN	MUTED	SILENCE
DEADEN	PEACEFUL	SOFT
GAGGED	PLACID	STILL
GENTLE	SECLUDED	TRANQUIL
HUSHED	SEDATE	WHISPER

"I... put my head under my pillow
and let the quiet put things where
they are supposed to be."

Stephen Chobsky

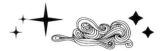

Clocks

```
L V Z B Z O Y D B X S S R
R E J R F W L I N D R B E
P W T O H A R Q Z E K T T
E E U N F D C A T W U Y A
T I I Z A O F E X R H G W
E G S E R M M T R S L O L
X H O D K O Y E D S D L L
D T M I N U T E S Z S O A
R S F O K D I A L A G R T
H M R A L A E R L S R O I
N H V H Y E K S R U O H G
C W G A O L F V K D G I I
J R V N O I T A R O C E D
L G D D J K I I S R Y O R
H P E S H J V Z A O W R T
```

ALARM	DIGITAL	MANTEL
BRONZE	FACE	MINUTES
CHRONOMETER	HANDS	REGULATOR
DECORATION	HOROLOGY	TURRET
DESK	HOURS	WATER
DIAL	KEY	WEIGHTS

"There is a time for many words, and there is also a time for sleep."

Homer

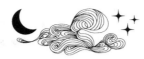

Words From the Letters in
"HOMO SAPIENS"

AMINO MASON

EMPHASIS NOISE

IMPASSE OMENS

INSEAM SHAMPOO

MANE   SIPHON

```
O  S  I  S  A  H  P  M  E
A  N  M  H  E  S  N  N  O
A  O  I  N  S  O  O  A  E
S  I  M  M  H  S  M  N  A
I  S  P  O  A  I  A  I  P
P  E  A  M  M  M  E  A  S
H  H  S  N  P  E  S  I  I
O  N  S  O  O  H  N  A  I
N  S  E  H  O  N  I  S  M
```

Food

COOKING MEAL

CUISINE NOURISH

DIET   RATIONS

FARE   SNACKS

GROCERIES SUSTAIN

```
G  H  S  I  R  U  O  N  A
R  O  L  A  E  M  C  S  G
O  B  R  V  S  U  U  N  E
C  L  F  A  I  S  I  S  E
E  D  Y  S  T  K  D  R  F
R  I  I  A  O  I  A  G  Y
I  N  I  O  E  F  O  E  E
E  N  C  T  I  R  N  N  R
S  B  P  S  N  A  C  K  S
```

"The main facts in human life are five:
birth, food, sleep, love and death."

E.M. Forster

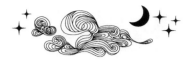

Food and Drink Diary

Make a record of what you ate and drank each day this week. Compare this with your sleep journal, what did you eat/drink when you slept well? What did you eat/drink when you slept badly? It is also important to make a note of the times you ate or drank each item in order to truly understand its effect on your sleep.

Use these prompts to help you remember what you have eaten and drunk today.

- Breakfast
- Lunch
- Dinner
- Snacks
- Drinks
- Did you consume caffeine or alcohol? How much?

<u>**Monday**</u>

....

....

<u>**Tuesday**</u>

....

....

<u>**Wednesday**</u>

....

....

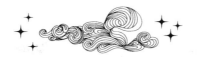

Thursday

....
....
....

Friday

....
....
....

Saturday

....
....
....

Sunday

....
....
....

Clever Things

```
M P K N S X P D E P T E C
C A L E R T E E R X F P U
T N E E K L Z A T G E E B
G H Z G O L H Y L Z D F T
L A N O I S S E F O R P A
T L H J E Q A T Y O E A T
D C V A X R G N T Q A C R
S M A R T O N E F Q D A E
B S D F A A G T A R Y D N
S R U N C E I E R S E E C
T L D I N O D P C V Q M H
I Y Y I R X P M I A R I A
L X U D M B U O E R I C N
A S A F S T U C Q Q K A T
T E T U T S A D E R S I R
```

ACADEMIC	COMPETENT	PROFESSIONAL
ADROIT	CRAFTY	READY
ALERT	DEFT	SCHOOLED
ARTFUL	DEVIOUS	SHARP
ASTUTE	GENIUS	SMART
CANNY	KEEN	TRENCHANT

"Go to bed smarter than when you woke up."

Charlie Munger

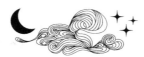

Ancient Writers

```
U R I U S L G T E R N O A
O N D E S A I T R A I T R
H A S L P A R G J D K A E
P P U O L E M S R N S L S
P N G P C Y T B X I J P P
A P N A V R Y R B P V E D
S D O I G A A P O Y B O B
O E L D A L A T O N I J E
S O S I C R A T E S I A K
A S E K S T E A E S H U U
R U S A G A T H I A S M S
L E O E D Y N I L P F O T
E M M S S I L L A G A V E
S E L O D C I C E R O I F
H A Q P H F R O T E L D A
```

AESOP	LIVY	PLATO
AGALLIS	LONGUS	PLINY
AGATHIAS	MOSES	SAPPHO
CICERO	OVID	SOCRATES
HESIOD	PETRONIUS	SOSICRATES
HOMER	PINDAR	VIRGIL

"The waking have one world in common; sleepers have each a private world of his own."

Heraclitus

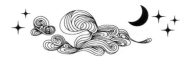

Mysterious

```
A  I  J  E  V  S  Y  O  N  B  L  O  S
L  N  Z  S  L  D  W  S  L  R  V  I  U
I  L  X  C  I  T  P  Y  R  C  I  I  O
R  A  E  L  C  N  U  D  A  V  N  P  I
E  U  V  E  X  S  I  B  A  E  A  C  T
G  S  W  R  T  M  A  S  X  R  I  D  I
N  U  E  L  I  A  Y  P  T  T  K  T  T
A  N  I  L  C  V  L  S  A  E  I  V  P
R  U  R  O  E  I  E  M  T  S  R  K  E
T  N  D  I  C  G  G  V  H  E  L  E  R
S  V  L  A  G  I  E  A  I  M  R  L  R
C  E  B  S  N  Z  D  N  D  T  Y  Y  U
D  L  R  E  E  Y  N  I  D  R  R  T  S
E  N  E  P  R  L  F  D  E  Z  R  U  H
C  C  I  T  S  Y  M  A  N  I  O  K  F
```

CRYPTIC	LEGEND	STRANGE
DARK	MYSTERY	SURREPTITIOUS
ENIGMATIC	MYSTIC	UNCLEAR
FURTIVE	MYTH	UNUSUAL
HIDDEN	SHADY	VEILED
INEXPLICABLE	SINISTER	WEIRD

"Bed is a bundle of paradoxes; we go to it with reluctance, yet we quit it with regret; and we make up our minds every night to leave it early, but we make up our bodies every morning to keep it late."

Charles Caleb Colton

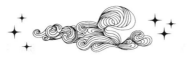

Nobel Peace Prize Winners

```
D M O Z O O O O A C D A J
L X Y T R I M B L E Y J O
U O U X D C U T B C O U H
E A N N A N A Z V E U O N
D R U S C D A S S N S B S
K U S H A O D R W R A O O
P I E S E Y K A B H F A N
N H V X A L I J M Y Z I S
M B B I T K N R T S A X I
H A E G E O H E O S I U R
I O A G E R O A R D T I L
Y X N T I E D A R A B L E
U E M U H N I I B O B B A
U T U T F A E D C P V I F
X K L R F L I X U L U F N
```

ADDAMS   ELBARADEI   SADAT
ANNAN   HUME   SAKHAROV
BEGIN   JOHNSON   TRIMBLE
BRANDT   SIRLEAF   TUTU
BUNCHE   LIU XIAOBO   YOUSAFZAI
CASSIN   MAATHAI   YUNUS
              RABIN

"Night is purer than day; it is better
for thinking and loving and dreaming.
At night everything is more intense,
more true. The echo of words that have
been spoken during the day takes
on a new and deeper meaning."

Elie Wiesel

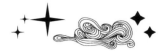

Words From the Letters in "ANDROMEDA"

ADDER
ADORNED
EON
MADRONE
MANOR

MOAN
MODERN
NOMAD
RANDOM
REMAND

```
E N E R D A M A M
E O R M N A D O R
D M O D E O M E O
D A E O R O D R N
N D O N D D N A A
A M E E A R A N M
O D R E M A N D O
O N M E D A D O E
A E N O R D A M O
```

68   Words From the Letters in "NIGHTMARE"

AGENT
ANTHEM
EMIGRANT
GERMAN
GRIME

MIRAGE
NIGHT
RANGE
TANGIER
TEAMING

```
G M G E M I R G N
N T E R A N G E N
I N T H I M I G G
M A H A T E M T E
A R A I N N H G R
E G I N A G A H M
T I E E I R I H A
R M E N I R G E N
A E A M T T R E R
```

"I have loved the stars too fondly to be fearful of the night."

Sarah Williams

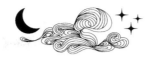

A Walk in the Woods

```
C A N Y L L O H O Y R R H
A V L I P Y V E F J O Y E
N W V P T H L E A R A N S
O Y Y T W L F H C R I B G
P R I M R O S E U D B H E
Y A Z K L U L D N B J M A
B G T I W B N L K I A B L
Y D A H H B A K I E L E H
E G B W S E C B R W R U L
E O A I T R F T A R O H O
X U A S E R S G I D E T L
C Y C E Z I G U Z D G S Y
A J P R C E Q A E N M E A
P E R C O S F E L P A M R
R E A K H W R L A P K Y R
```

BADGER	DEER	PATHS
BERRIES	FOLIAGE	PRIMROSE
BIRCH	HOLLY	SQUIRREL
CANOPY	IVY	STREAM
CREEPER	MAPLE	TRUNK
CROW	OWL	WILLOW

Sleep fact

Sleepwalking is a common parasomnia (sleep disorders involving abnormal movements) and may occur in up to 15% of people. Contrary to popular belief you should always wake a sleepwalker, it can be more dangerous to leave them sleeping, but be gentle!

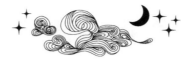

Don Quixote

```
B D E S T N A I G C G U F
I B F R H Q U I X A L B O
W S A O I W M L A S B D W
I P R E V U F V H T E C I
R S I A S R Q A B L V A N
E O A L I D H S O E W N D
A I C A G C R T E S C D M
E B R I N R H E P B H R I
N S M A N C I I H I I E L
I W M I V A W M D T V S L
C A R M C E N B S A A V S
L U C I N D A T B O L O F
U H N N F C D B E I R G G
D U C H E S S C U L Y U O
E P Q U I E O N A X I U Q
```

ANDRES	GIANTS	PILGRIMS
CASTLE	GOATHERDS	QUIXANO
CHIVALRY	HIDALGO	ROCINANTE
DUCHESS	HORSE	SQUIRE
DULCINEA	LA MANCHA	TOLEDO
FRIARS	LUCINDA	WINDMILLS

"Now, blessings light on him that first invented this same sleep! It covers a man all over, thoughts and all, like a cloak; it is meat for the hungry, drink for the thirsty, heat for the cold, and cold for the hot."

Miguel de Cervantes

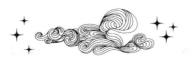

```
P V R H R I D V A N O B U
K F A J L Z A Z U V U I Q
S J P O Q Y J M M S B M N
J Y H P O B O N J H W R U
G B O D H I Q U A K E R S
A N R A M A D A N D G F T
H A A S Y A I V E K A A I
U C M D I C W S F O H S H
E I B S E N A T L E B A W
D L M W X M L F A V Z L W
Z G U R B C I S N O W I J
X N L Y H D Y B Y E I N X
Y A G E S H V T S R O S W
F O W M N A B A Q E V Z M
F S Y C F T K S G Z E L B
```

ANGLICAN	HOLI	RIDVAN
BELTANE	JUDAISM	SEDER
BODHI	LENT	TAOISM
DIWALI	OBON	WESAK
FASALI	QUAKERS	WHITSUN
HAJJ	RAMADAN	YULE

"It is better to sleep on things beforehand
than lie awake about them afterwards."

Baltasar Gracián

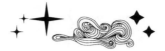

Sleep Disorders and Symptoms

```
P N D N A R C O L E P S Y
B C Y C Y X E L P A T A C
G S S E N L U F E K A W S
C M S I L U B M A N M O S
H N O L E R C E W O N A E
I P M R U D O N O D M N N
N T N X H N O D T O D B D
S H I U P C I T N O U S E
O S A A T N A D H S N D R
M D S U E T V S B O R A I
N W R S S I S E R U N E T
I I S S S E N I S W O R D
A C V S O M N I L O Q U Y
H Y P N A G O G I A H S F
R E C A T A T H R E N I A
```

APNOEA   ENURESIS   NSRED
BRUXISM   HYPNAGOGIA   SNORING
CATAPLEXY   INSOMNIA   SOMNAMBULISM
CATATHRENIA   MOODINESS   SOMNILOQUY
DROWSINESS   NARCOLEPSY   TIREDNESS
DYSSOMNIAS   NOCTURIA   WAKEFULNESS

"A little insomnia is not without its value in making us appreciate sleep, in throwing a ray of light upon that darkness."

Marcel Proust

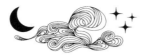

Kings and Queens

```
R R L A K L D L N Z C Q C
D V I C T O R I A M A R Y
G B U A U Y I I R U J A N
L X Z E L T T R C L X Z E
E O E J D F H G S H I E R
T Z D A I G R R D K A T Z
I N W N E K A E E B G R E
H A Y E E G H R D D Q D D
B M X Q Z T B A I I W R H
D I A X Q E U E R A N N E
F X T I D J E N R O O B N
F Y Y M L J A D A T L Z R
J W U H S L O M Q C O D Y
F N G K T D I H E L W A C
D E W D N D M W N S F E X
```

ALFRED	EDWARD	JANE
ANNE	EDWY	JOHN
CANUTE	EGBERT	MARY
CUTHRED	HAROLD	RICHARD
EDGAR	HENRY	VICTORIA
EDMUND	JAMES	WILLIAM

"One of the King George's of England—I forget which—once said that a certain number of hours' sleep each night—I cannot recall at the moment how many—made a man something, which for the time being has slipped my memory."

P.G. Wodehouse

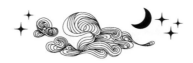

74   Words Containing "REST"

ARREST   RESTFUL
CREST   RESTORE
FAIREST   RESTRICT
FOREST   UNREST
INTEREST   WRESTLE

```
E T S E R T L T T
R P E I S U T S R
O A O E F S E E E
T F R T E R S R L
S C S R N E S E T
E E I U E N E T S
R A T R E S T N E
F O R E S T T I R
T C I R T S E R W
```

75   *A Connecticut Yankee in King Arthur's Court*

CAMELOT   MERLIN
CLARENCE   SANDY
ECLIPSE   SIR KAY
GALAHAD   THE BOSS
HANK   WARWICK

```
C C W S A N D Y M
V A L A D E A B E
E S M A R K G E R
Y S P E R W I N L
M O D I L E I D I
H B S N D O N C N
A E G M N V T C K
N H E S P I L C E
K T D A H A L A G
```

"I have never taken any exercise,
except sleeping and resting, and
I never intend to take any."

Mark Twain

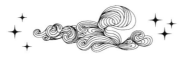

Doors

```
C R C D B T V H W Y F O A
O O N C N N S L I D I N G
F P M W S U W E S F C L Y
S B G P L P A N B B W S A
D N L F O L F A M T P S S
G O O A Y S V P A M W L T
N L O O S M I S J L G E W
I A D R L T S T E S K T R
T T D P F A P I E C B N P
A E F C L R S R O N D I O
T M O G S M A P O L L L P
O P W H O T E M V O O C H
R M W I C K E T E T F U U
E Y T I R U C E S I I Y Y
D H D E R V U O L E B M N
```

BIFOLD	JAMBS	ROTATING
BLAST-PROOF	LINTEL	SALOON
COMPOSITE	LOUVRED	SECURITY
DOOR FRAME	METAL	SLIDING
FLUSH	PANEL	STEEL
GLASS	POCKET	WICKET

In our dreams—Doors:

These may represent entering a new phase of
life. If they are open we are moving forward
with ease, if locked or difficult to open we may
be putting obstacles in front of ourselves.

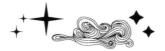

Jane Austen

```
S M R E L T O N E E G T Y
T R E N B Y E N V A S K A
E A A Y O H M E W H D M L
V G A R R T L E O R L R C
E I M I R Y S R R A K S S
N E N J N E E E D E A S R
T E L L B G F Y W L G M M
O K A I E E B D L R E I L
N A M N N E G E R S M T S
E H C M R O N R A A V H S
S Y I T S H R E O S W E C
M A R I A N N E H E M D A
Y A X M T D S O T A G M E
M N O T W A H C J S M H O
L A R D R O F A L E D E R
```

ALLENHAM

CHAWTON

DELAFORD

EDWARD
  FERRARS

ELINOR

EMMA

EVELYN

GEORGE

JAMES

LADY BERTRAM

LYME REGIS

MARIANNE

MR ELTON

MR WESTON

MRS CLAY

MRS SMITH

REGENCY

STEVENTON

"When I look out on such a night as this, I feel as if there could be neither wickedness nor sorrow in the world."

Jane Austen

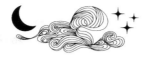

Dark Words

E	I	D	M	L	C	T	T	N	P	W	F	S
M	U	R	K	Y	M	E	W	W	D	S	N	S
S	E	Q	G	Y	J	I	C	O	N	U	M	E
E	S	K	A	L	N	G	D	D	B	R	S	N
N	W	H	C	P	O	N	F	N	E	V	L	K
E	I	O	A	A	O	O	W	U	I	I	V	R
V	P	G	D	D	L	P	M	S	P	G	B	A
E	N	B	H	A	E	B	A	A	T	L	H	D
N	E	S	R	T	H	D	H	H	A	L	I	T
T	C	B	N	W	T	S	G	C	M	B	A	U
I	L	T	D	N	S	I	K	E	T	Y	I	B
D	I	D	H	B	L	N	M	E	M	I	L	B
E	P	H	R	I	E	A	C	E	V	E	P	N
F	S	B	W	S	N	A	I	D	I	S	B	O
R	E	T	S	L	L	A	F	T	H	G	I	N

BLACKNESS   JET   OPAQUE
DARKNESS   MIDNIGHT   PITCH BLACK
DUSK   MURKY   SHADE
ECLIPSE   NIGHTFALL   SHADOW
EVENTIDE   NIGHT-TIME   SUNDOWN
GLOOM   OBSIDIAN   TWILIGHT

Sleep tip—A calm space:
A dark, quiet, cool room generally aids in both
falling asleep and remaining asleep.

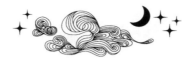

79   Sleeping Late

CATNAP   LOUNGE

DOZE   NAPPING

IDLE   SIESTA

LAZYBONES   SNOOZE

LIE IN   SPRAWL

```
A G M M E D L E L
T N E V E C F A O
S I E Z A Z Z H U
E P A T O Y O S N
I P N H B O P D G
S A R O S R N N E
P N N F A I L S N
O E G W L I E I N
S E L D I E H M C
```

80   Words From the Letters in "DAYBREAK"

BAKERY   DEAR

BARKED   DERBY

BREAK   RAKED

BYRE   READY

DARK   YEAR

```
A E A A K Y K A A
E A D Y Y E R Y B
B D E A R A R R Y
K K K B K R E E B
R B A R A A D K R
A Y R B D R A A E
D B E Y A E K Y D
B A K E R Y D E D
D K E B Y K R K D
```

"If you're going to do something tonight that you'll be sorry for in the morning, sleep late."

Henny Youngman

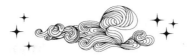

Sleep-related Films

```
A  X  S  L  A  I  N  M  O  S  N  I  E
N  S  I  O  S  U  O  I  D  I  S  N  I
R  I  D  R  P  P  A  P  R  I  K  A  W
E  B  N  A  T  I  S  I  V  S  O  S  D
K  U  U  C  B  A  T  L  I  B  O  N  R
L  L  O  S  E  R  M  R  U  S  D  P  E
A  C  B  A  F  P  A  E  L  M  A  A  N
W  T  L  M  D  L  T  Z  H  D  B  P  N
P  H  L  T  O  R  I  I  I  T  A  E  U
E  G  E  S  V  L  E  M  O  L  B  R  R
E  I  P  I  Y  L  N  A  C  N  E  H  E
L  F  S  R  N  E  W  I  M  Y  H  O  D
S  A  B  H  B  R  A  B  N  S  T  U  A
L  L  A  C  E  R  L  A  T  O  T  S  L
B  T  W  A  K  I  N  G  L  I  F  E  B
```

A CHRISTMAS CAROL

BLADE RUNNER

BRAZIL

DREAMS

FIGHT CLUB

INCEPTION

INSIDIOUS

INSOMNIA

PAPERHOUSE

PAPRIKA

SLEEPWALKER

SLUMBER

SOLARIS

SPELLBOUND

THE BABADOOK

THE MATRIX

TOTAL RECALL

WAKING LIFE

Sleep fact

More than 10% of people dream in black and white. It is more common in older people who grew up watching black and white televisions.

Gratitude

```
G N I V I G S K N A H T R
E R U T U F A Y F E H W D
E S A C K N O W L E D G E
A P P R E C I A T I O N W
E W L T N E M I L P M O C
S G V E Y G I U T F N F G
G G R M A E L C E D V K S
P N N A S S E A E N I G L
G D I I T P A R U N J D U
I G A V S E A N D T O O F
E R F E O S F N T H U W Y
P R R U R L E U S U E M O
M N A O U S I L L D P T J
B B U C S W V D B M C H V
M I E C N E I R E P X E O
```

ACKNOWLEDGE	EXPERIENCE	MUTUAL
APPRECIATION	FUTURE	PLEASANT
BLESSINGS	GRATEFUL	PRAISE
CARE	JOYFUL	RESPECT
COMPLIMENT	KINDNESS	THANKSGIVING
ENJOY	LOVING	WONDER

"End the day with gratitude. There is someone, somewhere that has less than you."

Zig Ziglar

Roads

```
C A T N E G D I R B S L G
C R Y E E S I R B D S G O
V I I A U H O R R N A N R
O T F N W U S I M H P I C
Y G E F T E V U T L Y S T
C J N E A E G D R W B S Y
O U R I Y R R A E F W O N
N N V S R L T C I F A R E
V C V I T E E C H R R C E
E T T D L O E T I A R B E
Y I B R T W N N A L N A F
A O I C A L T E I V B G C
N N H O O V W O O G I U E
C P A E V D E V A P N R P
E L E N N U T L L I A E P
```

BRIDGE
BYPASS
CARRIAGEWAY
CONVEYANCE
CROSSING
DRIVE

ENGINEERING
INTERCHANGE
JUNCTION
PAVED
PRIVATE
PUBLIC

ROUTE
STONE
SURFACE
TRAFFIC
TRAVEL
TUNNEL

In our dreams—Roads:

These can be indicative of our way forward, obstacles
in the road suggest difficulties on our chosen path,
turns in the road represent a change of direction,
and crossroads indicate decisions to be made.

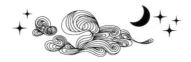

Philosophers

```
O E T E B B A D P R E A T
D E R R I D A L M F C C C
D M P N Y P U B N O R E L
P L A L O T L V N C I N I
E B T Y A A T F T C E E F
F P P R O T U H R A H S I
G A C T A C O G D M C C S
D H Z T I B R A F U S A E
A U E U B G Q Y Y S Z B A
P A S E A U R M W R T U U
P V S I I W E A E E D R
I G E N F L S L M T I D A
A H A V O F T U V S N H Y
H S E T O U H P A S C A L
F A P D B H I S A L V I K
```

APPIAH	DERRIDA	NIETZSCHE
AQUINAS	GRAMSCI	PASCAL
BUDDHA	HOBBES	PLATO
BUTLER	HUME	PLUTARCH
CAMUS	KANT	PTOLEMY
CONFUCIUS	LAO TZU	SENECA

"I am accustomed to sleep and in my dreams to imagine the same things that lunatics imagine when awake."

René Descartes

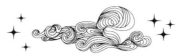

Assessing Your Bedtime Routine

Consider the following questions about your bedtime routine to see where it could improve.

How long before going to bed do you begin your bedtime routine?

....

....

What do you do to prepare for sleep? Do you take time out to clear your mind? Or spend time trying to get organized for the next day? Where your focus lies before attempting to settle down may impact your sleep.

....

....

....

How long before attempting to sleep do you switch off from all electronic devices?

....

Is your sleep environment calming? Is it tidy or cluttered? Do you have blackout blinds or does light filter in? etc.

....

How could you improve your routine?

....

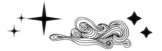

Feeling Confident

```
Y A A O S H B C H I P T E
D A S P I R I T E D F E S
L S O O A D T G E E Y N N
W S R V L S A L I T G A E
A U E O C R A L I B D C E
O R B Y U R E V G S B I C
Y E T O O B I F A S R T N
H D C M C T O O I E G Y E
E C N A I L E R F L E S D
S R E S O L U T E R P A I
I B O T G G N I R A D S F
O P T S U G B T S E A V N
P H P T U D N U W F M E O
D M S H R D Y D D R U C C
L Y W F U B C E R T A I N
```

ASSURED	COURAGE	POISE
BELIEF	DARING	POSITIVITY
BOLD	FEARLESS	RESOLUTE
BRAVERY	FORTITUDE	SELF-RELIANCE
CERTAIN	GUTSY	SPIRITED
CONFIDENCE	MORALE	TENACITY

In our dreams—Public nudity:

If we are seen this may represent a desire to reveal a part of ourselves. If we are alone this likely represents a wish for freedom of expression.

```
C O D C V D R C A H S H S
G N A E A E O M F T B T D
L B N O L R R O E T I V I
R U T O S B A R W B B S G
T R A B A W R V B D S S A
M G H D L E N A A A L P R
U O G R F T R E L N E I O
R E N A M O W R E H S A W
R E H O V E F I B F A W I
W S T A O T S V A H E R N
I H I T H M E E N G W E G
P R I S O N X R Q N V P B
N L Y L T R O P U L U V O
F V E W C H F N E S T E A
T E U Q A R F W T A R O T
```

BANQUET	MR BADGER	RIVER
CARAVAN	MR TOAD	ROWING BOAT
FERRETS	OTTER	STOATS
FOXES	PORTLY	WASHERWOMAN
GAOLER	PRISON	WEASELS
MOLE	RABBITS	WILD WOOD

"Dark and deserted as it was, the night was full of small noises, song and chatter and rustling, telling of the busy little population who were up and about...through the night till sunshine should fall on them at last and send them off to their well-earned repose."

Kenneth Grahame

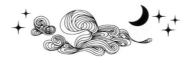

Feeling Snug

```
C O Y A W A E D I H C R R
S H O O Z E H G B O R E G
E L Z Z U N B U N D L E W
Z U N V L U D T L A O M W
O F H L R U E E X C O Z D
O R B R M N X E R U C W E
N M O I T S D U S U T Y U
S W E O T O A B R L C P E
R E T L E H S L U Y E E O
A A F E H O U F A L H A S
E T O S E P S Y D C T C E
S T S F S S E D B W M E O
O R A E I N U T G H R F Z
R S W L N C V U U P A U E
M A B U R G T A M T W L G
```

BLISSFUL	DOZE	RELAXED
BUNDLE	HIDEAWAY	SAFE
BURROW	LUXURY	SECURE
CONTENT	NEST	SHELTER
CUDDLE	NUZZLE	SNOOZE
CURL UP	PEACEFUL	WARMTH

Sleep tip—Comfort is key:

A good mattress has a life expectancy of 9 to 10 years, yours might have outlived its efficiency.

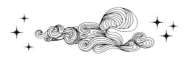

Excerpt: *Wynken, Blynken, and Nod*
Eugene Field

```
W A V E S A L B G L I D N
D R P O R A G N A S W I I
E E R H T O O N L H H A G
I V P S T S E U E S W S H
R I Y S R K F R L I G H T
C R E A N I E R N W M R G
C A T Y T V W D G O I N G
A S L U E C E Y O C O M E
S B A R A L A N N L E N G
N E T S I L V E R K O P N
B N T A H W L V O D E L I
M E S D L O G E C F I N R
L A U G H E D R K V I A R
D E L F F U R W E D A S E
D R A E F A N E D O O W H
```

Wynken, Blynken, and Nod one night
   Sailed off in a wooden shoe–
Sailed on a river of crystal light,
   Into a sea of dew.
"Where are you going, and what do you wish?"
   The old moon asked of the three.
"We have come to fish for the herring fish
That live in this beautiful sea;
Nets of silver and gold have we!"
      Said Wynken,
      Blynken,
      And Nod.

The old moon laughed and sang a song,
   As they rocked in the wooden shoe,
And the wind that sped them all night long
   Ruffled the waves of dew.
The little stars were the herring fish
   That lived in that beautiful sea–
"Now cast your nets wherever you wish–
   Never afeard are we!"
So cried the stars to the fishermen three:
      Wynken,
      Blynken,
      And Nod.

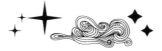

The Science of Sleep

```
E G N I N O T A L E M K I
A R E D Y C D N H Y R H U
T A U A T E H T S E R H M
R C I H L D S T J E S Y I
A T E T Q M A C G B E P C
N I A U A G I A H P L A R
S V I E E N W L G W D M O
I E R S P A R G E R N E S
T D N Y K P M C T B I M L
I Y H E Y C H G A P P O E
O O N U L Y T M L B S R E
N E E R S M Y E C U L Y P
D P U G N I H T A E R B L
W C C T C I R C A D I A N
N I N O T O R E S O N I N
```

ACTIVE	DREAMS	RHYTHM
ALPHA	HYPNIC JERK	SEROTONIN
AWAKENED	MELATONIN	SPINDLES
BREATHING	MEMORY	STAGES
CIRCADIAN	MICROSLEEP	THETA
DELTA	QUIET	TRANSITION

Sleep fact

Super sleepers require only four to five hours
sleep compared to the average of six to eight
hours that most people require, but it is incredibly
rare and likely due to a genetic anomaly.

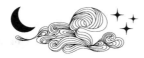

Stars and Constellations

```
G  E  M  P  R  O  Y  S  N  L  L  C  S
C  T  O  Y  C  E  Y  U  Y  O  S  G  C
A  D  A  A  I  F  A  R  Y  U  I  N  I
N  S  R  Q  A  L  A  E  S  V  B  R  W
C  D  E  R  U  S  I  A  S  E  D  P  O
E  C  I  R  U  A  G  P  U  Q  U  A  N
R  E  Y  R  A  E  R  S  H  U  I  F  D
S  I  U  E  P  T  U  I  C  E  R  E  R
E  A  E  B  D  I  N  R  U  W  I  D  A
T  N  A  O  P  V  Y  A  I  S  A  G  H
E  O  G  R  I  G  E  L  H  P  L  M  P
C  M  O  S  B  E  F  O  P  T  I  Y  L
O  C  S  E  C  S  I  P  O  P  U  E  A
S  G  E  M  I  N  I  T  A  U  Q  A  M
Y  E  A  D  E  M  O  R  D  N  A  L  T
```

ALPHARD	CANCER	PEGASUS
ANDROMEDA	DRACO	PISCES
ANTARES	GEMINI	POLARIS
AQUARIUS	LYRA	RIGEL
AQUILA	OPHIUCHUS	SCORPIUS
ARIES	ORION	TAURUS

"I like the night. Without the dark,
we'd never see the stars."

Stephenie Meyer

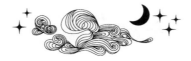

Extreme Sports

```
H G N I T I U S G N I W A
A D N S M O T O C R O S S
T E G I Y B A E Y N I N G
I E N V D P G E H V B K U
P R I Y Z I P L I N I N G
A A L E F I L A F T C G D
R F I S C C F G E A N N U
K T E L K E I S G I B I I
O I S O R Y U E B N F L R
U N B R O R D R G L A O O
R G A U F I O I U H P H N
E T E I V Z A V V G T T M
A A N I E H R N E I C O A
T G N I N O Y N A C N P N
S G B O U L D E R I N G P
```

ABSEILING   IRONMAN   SKYDIVING
BOULDERING   KITESURFING   VIA FERRATA
CAGE DIVING   MOTOCROSS   WING SUITING
CANYONING   PARKOUR   ZIP LINING
HANG GLIDING   POTHOLING   ZORBING
                   RAFTING

In our dreams—Edge of a cliff:

This may indicate we are facing danger and
need to make a decision, especially one that
involves risk and facing the unknown.

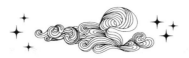

The Brontë Sisters

```
R Y E R G S E N G A L F P
A E M L O C L Y B E F A H
H H R Y O M U W U I T T X
S H I R L E Y L L R R E A
L N E W U T D C I O A O F
R U F R W C H C W E R Y R
E F C W Y T K A R P D U I
G N P Y A E H G P I O S A
C S N E S D E O H D O V F
N C H A B N E N V I W G S
M E L O B M O L A F K M R
A C L P S W Y W E J C W M
R N A E D Y L L E N O G P
I B R D H B R E M I L Y B
A O F R E T S E H C O R O
```

ADELE	HEATHCLIFF	MRS FAIRFAX
AGNES GREY	HELEN	NELLY DEAN
ANNE	JANE EYRE	PATRICK
CURRER	LOCKWOOD	POEMS
EMILY	LUCY SNOWE	ROCHESTER
HAWORTH	MARIA	SHIRLEY

"I love the silent hour of night,
For blissful dreams may then arise,
Revealing to my charmed sight
What may not bless my waking eyes!"

Anne Brontë

Fears

```
R A W R A E L C U N I S H
M E C Y S D W O R C H N E
M A K C O L D A G E A O G
H O W K I D A D A R G S S
F O R G R D A G B S N I T
S T R A N G E R S A S O A
D C O S E D W N K D P P K
G E S L E I C E T N E O E
L U A G A S S M P S E P S
N E C T R E L Y Z M D S F
H T P E H A A C L O W N S
T S T O G S M N U A T E O
F A M I N E I T M E S A M
W L I G H T N I N G A T I
E R A S E C A P S N E P O
```

ACCIDENTS	DISEASE	OPEN SPACES
ANIMALS	FAMINE	POISON
CLOWNS	HORSES	SNAKES
CROWDS	LIGHTNING	SPEED
DARKNESS	NUCLEAR WAR	STRANGERS
DEATH	OLD AGE	WATER

In our dreams—Running away:

This likely indicates a fear or inability to do something.

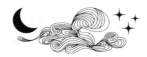

94   In Nature

ANIMAL   LIFE
COUNTRY   PASTORAL
FAUNA   RURAL
FLORA   SCENERY
LANDSCAPE   WORLD

```
E P A C S D N A L
S A N U A F Y A O
Y N D B N R R P E
R P A S T O R A L
E U P N L U N P I
N F U F R I O N F
E O R A M U V F E
C L L A W O R L D
S N L P L Y G A G
```

95   Words From the Letters in "RESTORED"

DESERT   SORE
ERRED   STEER
ORDER   STEREO
RESORT   TERSE
RESTED   TREES

```
T D E T S E R D T
R E E R R R O E R
R E O E R E T S R
E E S R E E E E S
R S E O O E D R T
O R T R R R T T E
T E E O E T D D E
T T S E T O O E R
E S E E R T R D R
```

"Tired Nature's sweet restorer, balmy sleep!
He, like the world, his ready visit pays
Where fortune smiles; the
wretched he forsakes."

Edward Young

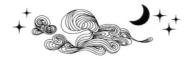

The Bedroom

```
A L M P P N C L W M F W B
C B A A E I S L H W P M R
H C S M I G L T O B T N F
E L T S P H A L E T W O I
S O E G N T D R O E H T C
T S R Y M S U A O W H E U
H E W T W T E E M T S S S
R T F Y A A O V A L S A H
V F S C E N W T T F R H I
A W Y E M D A E T O F O O
N E N S U I T E R O P C N
I G O T U G F R E W M H S
T A B S N V I B S C Y A I
Y T T B V M N S S A D I N
W A R E T R O F M O C R T
```

CHAIR	EN SUITE	NIGHTSTAND
CHEST	GUEST	OTTOMAN
CLOSET	LAMP	PILLOWS
CLOTHES	MASTER	SHEETS
COMFORTER	MATTRESS	STORAGE
CUSHIONS	MIRROR	VANITY

Sleep tip—Beds are for sleeping:

Help your brain to associate bed with sleep by only using it for sleep. Do not work, watch TV, or use your phone in bed and your mind will find it easier to switch off.

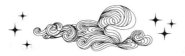

Famous Scots

```
S  R  O  G  E  R  G  C  M  N  T  W  H
N  B  B  O  P  S  R  C  P  T  R  O  M
R  O  Y  G  R  C  P  P  A  R  I  F  D
U  P  S  D  O  O  W  W  P  M  U  Y  D
B  T  I  N  C  T  M  H  T  I  M  S  L
S  E  A  R  E  T  M  C  A  V  O  Y  A
E  M  U  H  S  V  P  N  M  R  C  P  N
T  H  W  A  R  B  E  L  T  A  H  B  O
M  B  E  A  H  E  O  T  R  U  W  H  D
U  T  A  N  L  H  L  N  S  W  C  R  C
R  C  L  R  S  L  E  T  C  Y  I  T  A
R  A  Y  I  R  G  A  R  U  A  Y  I  M
A  O  H  A  I  I  E  C  B  B  D  D  U
Y  C  P  E  B  I  E  P  E  I  A  D  E
I  D  O  T  Y  L  L  O  N  N  O  C  F
```

BAIRD	CONNOLLY	MURRAY
BARRIE	HUME	SCOTT
BURNS	MACDONALD	SMITH
BUTLER	MCAVOY	STEVENSON
CARNEGIE	MCGREGOR	WALLACE
CHISHOLM	MUIR	WATT

"Sleep the night that knows not breaking,
Morn of toil, nor night of waking."

Sir Walter Scott

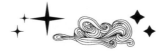

```
R E N N I P S N L R A U L
S E B O N I A A E T E R R
W I N H N R O B N E A M U
E T T E W G B V R A L T Y
O T N H M U E R D P I A G
R C A U L Y R W E U S U B
P L E B W O L V H L S R G
E T L S G E T C P G L K M
S O I T E O H P R B H I Y
P O H R L Y P I E R L A K
Y T C I I V G L V N C U B
G H P P A H U S E Q A N E
M E W E T G S D U S L T L
Y D I D A V A Q U I T A U
S R O T C E H I S V E U C
```

BALEEN	DUSKY	PYGMY
BELUGA	GUIANA	RIGHT
BLUBBER	HECTOR'S	SPINNER
BLUE	KILLER	STRIPED
CHILEAN	NARWHAL	TOOTHED
CLYMENE	PILOT	VAQUITA

Sleep fact

Whales and dolphins only fall half asleep, each side
of their brain takes it in turns waking and sleeping
so that they can continue to surface to breathe.

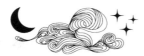

Dr Seuss Characters

```
F R C S R S O H A W L G H
F I I T I Y J S G I N T W
O N R H A O O O K I B M T
K G A E H K J P L O A L A
I H L C G N C I I I O L A
D C A A S D E I M D U Z A
A N R T D G R A W E D B H
L I I I S F S A N D R E E
V R S N I S I O S B I N I
D G T T H M T S L I O H C
A E O H W R A O H G L L T
L H T E O U O Y N Y A A F
V T R H N G H I U R S G R
A A O A S N H S K G T G U
L W H T T T H E L O R A X
```

ALI SARD	GUY-AM-I	THE GRINCH
BLOOGS	HORTON	THE LORAX
CLARK	JOJO	THIDWICK
GEILING	SAM-I-AM	THING ONE
GHAIR	SIR ALARIC	VLAD
GLAD FISH	THE CAT IN THE HAT	VLADIKOFF
		ZOOKS

"A yawn is quite catching,
you see. Like a cough.
It takes just one yawn to
start other yawns off."

Dr Seuss

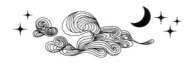

Exploration and Discovery

```
T S P I H S D R A H E L E
G A W I R O M E R E O D S
V O Y A G E G E S A X E X
N J I P M V A N C Y I E S
S E Z J V A E F O L T L A
L A A R I O P D P C Q O E
L J C Q D J L P J V E P S
A I I Q V N U Q I D S H H
F T R I O S T C A N P T T
R H F Z R R T R S A G U U
E M A Y A O T H L O Q O O
T M D I R E C T I O N S S
A E L I T E L G N U J U V
W S A W D I W H P E D A I
N O Y N A C D N A R G G U
```

AFRICA	HARDSHIPS	TRADE
AMAZON	JUNGLE	TRAILS
CONGO	MAPPING	UJIJI
DIRECTION	SOUTH POLE	VICTORIA
GRAND CANYON	SOUTH SEAS	VOYAGE
HAITI	SUPPLIES	WATERFALLS

In our dreams—Immobility:

This may indicate we have created circumstances which are beginning to make us feel trapped, we should be still while we choose our way forward.

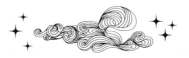

Novelists

```
J H I C K S E M A J W G S
L F L P J C R R E D I W U
E P E V E S W E A L I M T
T C O N A N D O Y L E T M
N A S D H S C L D A G H M
A T A R C H E R D B S A N
M M U U M A C A R E I C D
S D E R S V D M A S R K A
M S Y O E M I C H E N E R
T A R Y R T U J N W F R N
F R A N C I S D I E W A O
I Y S H S U E R E L D Y C
W N E I K L O T O L V U T
S L U A L L O E O F E T A
L O S O B H Y B I G S O N
```

ADAMS	FRANCIS	RENDELL
ARCHER	JAMES	SAYERS
AUDEN	LEASOR	SEWELL
CONAN DOYLE	MANTEL	SWIFT
CONRAD	MICHENER	THACKERAY
FORSTER	MITCHELL	TOLKIEN

"A ruffled mind makes a restless pillow."

Charlotte Brontë

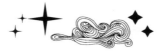

Emotions

```
V M A R T U Y M G E X R D
O Z P P S K S P Z F S U R
H C I R Z H A L E E X Z E
W J T X O X W E O A H E A
P C Y C T Y C R H R C X D
U E K N T S W C A C B E C
C O N S T E R N A T I O N
D T O A S Y R Z J G H R Q
I U S D U T P R K W Y E U
S Y S N G A E A O H Q D A
M X A E S M Q R M R M N L
A C G S I Y R J G R H O A
Y G I S D O D X K E V W R
P O Y U S B Z K H E R B M
N A K C U J G F N M K O P
```

ALARM
CONSTER-
   NATION
DISGUST
DISMAY
DREAD
ECSTASY

FEAR
LOVE
PASSION
PEACE
PITY
REGRET

SADNESS
SHOCK
SORROW
TERROR
WONDER
WRATH

"The best bridge between despair and hope is a good night's sleep."

E.J. Cossman

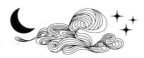

"DAY" Words

```
C A V S A D G E K N W E S
R O V F L O W E R R S L Y
D E F D N F S I C A O A B
H I P A M R O H E E L W S
W C I P T Q U L I I X W S
O Q T S I O E T G F I K E
D L Y A C R N H E B T E N
L R Y R W S T E U R T E D
A R E S E S C G M N D W N
T O E A W G A H J E S E I
I F T D M O R A O J N H L
P U A I A E R U R O I T B
S N S U A R R E S T L F I
O F E F B S T S E R F O T
H T N E M G D U J F O R E
```

BLINDNESS	OF JUDGMENT	SHIFT
DREAMER	OF REST	SURGERY
FLOWER	OF THE WEEK	TRADER
HOSPITAL	RELEASE	TRIPPER
LIGHT	RETURN	WATCH
OF ATONEMENT	SCHOOL	WORK

"Finish each day before you begin the next, and interpose a solid wall of sleep between the two. This you cannot do without temperance."

Ralph Waldo Emerson

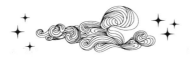

105 Words From the Letters in "DORMANCY"

ACRONYM DRAM
ADORN MANOR
ARMY MORDANCY
CANDY RANDOM
CORN YARD

```
C M C M R D N D R
N R O D A D M O R
Y R N R C O O O M
M A R D D D N Y C
R N R N C A N O N
A A A N R O N A M
Y R R O R N Y C D
N O N C A N D Y Y
C D A C N M C N R
```

106 Laughter

FUNNY HOWL
GIGGLE MIRTH
GLEE SHRIEK
GUFFAW SNORT
HAHA TICKLED

```
T I N S M E N A C
W E Y A C S F D A
A L E L H U O E T
F G P E N A K L R
F G U N L E H K O
U I Y H I G T C N
G G O R U O R I S
O W H R E L I T E
L S P G O E M I D
```

"A good laugh and a long sleep are
the two best cures for anything."

Irish Proverb

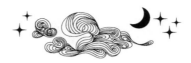

The Weather

```
R A G C R O O B D C V Y S
F D L C S C Y R L S T U W
J R O E N U J I R S L A B
E O O A D G M X I T T M S
G U M N A A Q M R O T S E
N G Y P T S H Y A A R I B
O H E E M A Q U T R I A S
O T N A O H L U T R Y N G
S T E C S D G S A A A S Y
N E Y Y P A R W Y L I H S
O Y V R H E S I N S L O C
M B H E E D M N Z P T W C
C L E A R Y Y D L Z C E I
A M E F E E K Y C E L R M
M S T R O M E R A E S E P
```

ATMOSPHERE	FRONTAL SYSTEM	SHOWER
CHART	GLOOMY	SQUALL
CLEAR	MISTY	STORM
CLIMATE	MONSOON	SULTRY
DRIZZLE	RAINY	SUMMARY
DROUGHT	SEVERE	WINDY

"A cool breeze stirred my hair at that moment, as the night wind began to come down from the hills, but it felt like a breath from another world."

Francis Marion Crawford

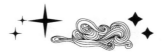

Activity Diary

Make a record of your activity levels each day.
Be sure to record the times at which any activities were
undertaken during the day. Compare this to your sleep
journal to see what effect your activity during the day
has on your sleep at night.

Ask yourself these questions:
- Did you exercise today?
- How much physical activity did you
take outside of exercise?
- How mentally busy did you feel?
- Did you leave a lot of tasks incomplete?
- Did you work?
- What other activities/hobbies did you engage in?

Monday

....

....

Tuesday

....

....

Wednesday

....

....

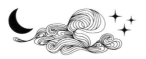

Thursday

....

....

....

Friday

....

....

....

Saturday

....

....

....

Sunday

....

....

....

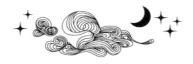

Astrology

```
U S P P S E R A O T E P A
R A T F R E M A G R E G W
A S E T A E A I R S I G N
R E A R T H D R I M O O N
B E P C S D U I V L D L B
I R A O T I I R C V E A D
L P E D C A U E L T K J T
R R F S I S Q H S E I B W
J E L E A N O C I S C O I
T C X H U Y G R C U I T N
A N B S E I L A O O L L S
U A R I E S I Y H H E T Y
R C C F E D H G H E L Y E
U S E B O S T G H W E G R
S A K Z O D A W N E S T A
```

AIR SIGN	HOROSCOPE	STARS
ARCHER	HOUSE	TAURUS
ARIES	LIBRA	TWINS
CANCER	MOON	VIRGO
EARTH	PREDICTION	WHEEL
FISHES	READING	ZODIAC

"There is a dead spot in the night, that coldest, blackest time when the world has forgotten evening and dawn is not yet a promise. A time when it is far too early to arise, but so late that going to bed makes small sense."

Robin Hobb

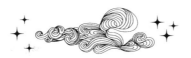

Human Characters

```
Q T T S I M I T P O D J P
E D N M L T H P O P G N D
A H B A B B L E R P T R M
S B O H D U L S R S E L I
A A D T R E R N I E O O S
D R D K H B P T B A T P E
I B B A G E A R F C I I R
S A A H Y M A E E T U P C
T R L O G D R D H D W I G
E I L O Q K R C F P A Y A
V A D L C S T E O M J E Q
A N K I L J I J A N L L L
N P E G L N R K L M M G S
K H L A D N A V N L E A Z
F Y O N R E M R A H C R N
```

BABBLER	HERETIC	MISER
BARBARIAN	HOOLIGAN	ODDBALL
CHARMER	HOTHEAD	OPTIMIST
CON MAN	KNAVE	PEDANT
DAYDREAMER	LEADER	SADIST
DOGMATIST	LOAFER	VANDAL

Sleep fact

The foetal position—lying on your side with your
legs curled up—is the most common sleep position.
Some studies report that our sleeping position
can reveal things about our personality.

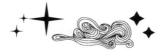

Things We Love

```
E  T  A  L  O  C  O  H  C  N  P  W  J
B  D  T  M  I  C  J  U  T  U  H  W  S
G  U  L  Y  R  E  S  T  Z  F  Z  J  L
M  G  T  N  O  I  C  Z  Q  C  K  E  L
C  N  F  T  S  L  L  A  H  E  Y  L  E
I  I  R  Q  E  E  D  I  R  N  D  L  B
S  C  I  T  S  R  L  M  N  O  P  Y  H
U  N  E  E  I  D  F  A  O  O  L  X  G
M  A  D  Z  R  U  R  L  E  V  Q  S  I
I  D  O  E  R  G  R  T  I  D  I  Q  E
E  T  N  F  J  X  R  F  T  E  D  E  L
L  Y  I  E  A  Y  Z  W  K  C  S  C  S
S  G  O  D  T  O  H  I  N  P  U  K  H
G  B  N  V  F  G  N  I  H  G  U  A  L
D  C  S  H  C  A  E  B  E  H  T  I  B
```

BUTTERFLIES	FRUIT	OLD MOVIES
CAROLS	GRANNY	POETRY
CHILDREN	HOT DOGS	PUZZLES
CHOCOLATE	JELLY	ROSES
DANCING	LAUGHING	SLEIGH BELLS
FRIED ONIONS	MUSIC	THE BEACH

"The way to a more productive,
more inspired, more joyful life
is getting enough sleep."

Arianna Huffington

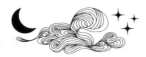

People Who Have Held Guinness World Records

```
E P E R C E M S D A S O N
B L G S I D E T I H W F I
A R H W F F R G R A N D E
U E O O Y U V A G N C U A
M B J A F R V O Y O R L R
G E W O N M L E S T D A E
A O M N H A C E M R T A D
R T A R N N S T I A N R M
T S D L E E S N C P E M O
N H D R S B B O C P M S N
E T W R I W P F N A L T D
R A O E F F I L C D A R C
L C B I L T W F W A C O E
S E U U E P R L T F D N W
R N W O L D A W F T V G F
```

ALDRIN	FURMAN	REDMOND
ARMSTRONG	GRANDE	SCORSESE
BAUMGARTNER	JOHNSON	STOEBERL
BIEBER	LAWRENCE	SWIFT
BOWIE	PARTON	WADLOW
CALMENT	RADCLIFFE	WHITE

Sleep fact

Randy Gardner remained awake for 11 days in 1964—it is disputed as to whether this record has been broken— it is not recommended, consequences of extreme sleep deprivation can be dire and include death.

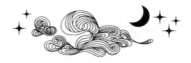

Peanuts

```
S Y L L A S L Y P O O N S
A P R O I P H O S T O R D
Y D I B E E T H O V E N A
U L E K G N E P G I P T R
W L S I E I E C E Y I A N
O A U E R U V E V L M D I
O B E C D F Y S H H V V L
D E F O Y R H U T I P I K
S S R Y M E N O O L M Y N
T A B V R C S L I N U S A
O B Y M C S E Y C T W C R
C S Y D I T E I C R A M F
K G L M N F G A R P A Y R
N A E J Y G G E P U E R A
B Y O N R E D E O R H C S
```

BASEBALL	LUCY	SCHROEDER
BEETHOVEN	MARCIE	SHERMY
EUDORA	MISS OTHMAR	SNOOPY
FRANKLIN	PEGGY JEAN	SPIKE
FRIEDA	PIG-PEN	VIOLET
LINUS	SALLY	WOODSTOCK

"Sometimes you lie in bed at night, and you don't have a single thing to worry about... That always worries me!"

Charles M. Schulz

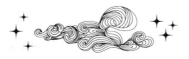

Lost

```
H D E L T T E S N U I H T
I P D I A L S I M M D N M
D R U E I U W A O I E S P
D E B Z P S B V O S R U E
E O T B Z H S B B S E N R
N C M N H L Y A T I H C P
I C O P E T E R N N T O L
N U V N W I A D F G E N E
V P A L F Y R F C E T S X
I I N T E U O O A V N C E
S E I D N E S D S S U I D
I D S N S A R E H I R O S
B C H H O I A P D Y D U C
L R E B F R O O T L E S S
E H D T G N I R E D N A W
```

ABSENT	MISLAID	STRAYED
ADRIFT	MISSING	UNCONSCIOUS
CONFUSED	PERPLEXED	UNSETTLED
DISORIENTED	PREOCCUPIED	UNTETHERED
HIDDEN	PUZZLED	VANISHED
INVISIBLE	ROOTLESS	WANDERING

In our dreams—Being/feeling lost:

Whether emotionally, physically, or spiritually this may show we have lost the ability to make clear decisions.

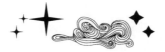

Quilting

```
P A O T K B E S T I N G N
C P F C N E E D L E S U D
I P O N R G B S H P E S A
R L N F N E C I I M T A S
B I O C C I K L N M Q U O
A Q T R S O C R R D U G M
F U T S L R F P A H I I R
S E O S E V O L G M L N A
C R E D T N I H A S T V G
S O N G O I T R N Y E R N
E O T S I U T H G E E E O
W Y E T T F B C R E M R L
C E E A O R M L H E H U S
T R A P U N T O E E A B D
G G N I T S A B E T S D A
```

APPLIQUE	FABRIC	QUILT
BASTING	GLOVES	SCISSORS
BINDING	LAYERS	STITCHES
BLOCK	LONGARM	THREAD
COTTON	MARKER	TRAPUNTO
DOUBLET	NEEDLES	WONDER CLIPS

"If you can't sleep, then get up
and do something instead of lying
there worrying. It's the worry that
gets you, not the lack of sleep."

Dale Carnegie

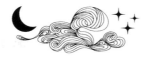

REM Songs

```
R E P E E L S Y A D N W M
V T D R I V E M A E O E I
D A H T S E P L E T I N V
S U P E R M A N R B C D M
N E M N O L L A F T I E A
A A G D B N E T S L P L N
N L M D N H E U L R S L O
I P G W Y A L I A S U G N
M D T M O R T D L Y S E T
A H H O E L I S Y O P E H
L O S D N O L A H U V U E
D O N F S G D O T N U E M
I A T O V D U E H W E H O
W H N U A U G E I H A A O
H G N B S L T O A E E S N
```

ANIMAL
BAD DAY
DAYSLEEPER
DRIVE
FALL ON ME
GET UP

HOLLOW MAN
LOTUS
MAN ON THE MOON
OH MY HEART
RADIO SONG
STAND

SUPERMAN
SUSPICION
THE ONE I LOVE
TONGUE
WANDERLUST
WENDELL GEE

Sleep fact

We sleep in 90-minute cycles, each cycle contains REM (dream) sleep even if only briefly, meaning we all dream multiple times a night.

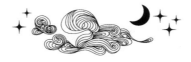

Sleepy Words

```
D L E S Y T D A V E R V E
N R B T E S R E N G A I F
V S I I N E R E N E R E S
S A U F Z E D I U O E T N
G Q U I T S T R P E B A S
O E E B A O T N R S M N E
O Z P L E P F C O D U R N
D O E P T E R F N C L E I
N O T B T R E A X D S B L
I N P E E L S L B A B I C
G S G L M L T I E G L H E
H D S D V B F U I M F E R
T O O M L I U Q N A R T R
F E I Z P I L L O W E R S
H A R G E E M S E C A E P
```

CONTENT	PILLOW	SANDMAN
DOZE	QUIET	SERENE
DRIFT OFF	RECLINE	SLEEP
GOODNIGHT	RELAX	SLUMBER
HIBERNATE	REPOSE	SNOOZE
PEACE	RESTFUL	TRANQUIL

"Fatigue is the safest sleeping draught."

Virginia Woolf

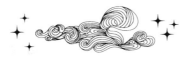

National Forests of the USA

```
S O E E D A L O B I C L E
I I L D I F E M T L R U S
R R L T I X E D A N I E E
G A L L A T I N R N O T R
I Y O D A R O D L E G T D
A D E N O H T O H S R E A
N E Z P E R C E A W A Y P
E L D B R H A N N E N A S
T D R V U R J F O S D P O
O M U G R U M F S M E D L
O G A E A U Y A E R L O G
K C I N E N G A R E H A E
H S L A E N O H S O H S S
N A E I O P A S B O I S E
N I A T N U O M E T I H W
```

BOISE	KOOTENAI	SAN JUAN
CHUGACH	LOS PADRES	SHOSHONE
CIBOLA	NEZ PERCE	SIERRA
DIXIE	PAYETTE	TONGASS
ELDORADO	RIO GRANDE	TONTO
GALLATIN	SALMON-CHALLIS	WHITE MOUNTAIN

In our dreams—Forests:

These are often related to our emotional self
and our understanding of our own natures.

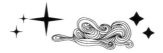

117 Words From the Letters in "BEAUTIFUL"

ALBEIT FAULT
BEFIT FAUTEUIL
BELT FIBULAE
BLUE FLUTE
FABLE TUBULE

T	E	L	U	B	U	T	L	I
U	F	E	A	L	U	B	I	F
A	T	E	T	U	U	L	B	A
L	B	T	I	A	I	U	A	U
B	E	U	F	E	A	E	U	T
E	T	L	E	A	B	L	B	E
I	A	F	B	E	U	I	E	U
T	A	U	L	A	A	L	U	I
A	U	T	B	I	F	E	T	L

118 Words That Come Before or After "BODY"

BUILDER GUARDS
BUSY SOME
CHECK SUIT
DOGS SURFING
EVERY WORKS

D	E	T	E	B	E	R	A	F
I	R	O	E	V	L	G	B	G
W	P	M	E	G	E	H	U	N
R	O	R	S	S	E	R	S	I
S	D	R	A	U	G	L	Y	F
L	E	A	K	F	I	O	S	R
C	Y	V	N	S	H	T	D	U
A	C	H	E	C	K	S	O	S
R	E	D	L	I	U	B	E	B

"It was a night so beautiful that
your soul seemed hardly able to
bear the prison of the body."

W. Somerset Maugham

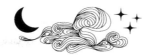

US States

```
W D M E X O Z H T T V Y G
I A A A I G H C N K G V C
S R Z H I T V J O F N A H
C M O G E N C O M F I N A
O U O X J E E Y R I M A W
N A A N C W S J E D O I A
S S B F T H N X V A Y D I
I O N E V A D A A H W N I
N N K V T M N A M O O I H
A Z T L N P S A L G C A P
N W M N A S F A E A T G A
Y F O F C H Q R S U S H P
A D J I K I O N O N A K R
Y V E F C R C M X U A Y A
W T J R H E H N A Z L K V
```

ALASKA
HAWAII
IDAHO
INDIANA
IOWA
KANSAS

MAINE
MONTANA
NEVADA
NEW
    HAMPSHIRE
OHIO
OKLAHOMA

OREGON
TEXAS
UTAH
VERMONT
WISCONSIN
WYOMING

Sleep fact

Dakota has some unusual sleeping laws. In South Dakota it is illegal to lie down and fall asleep in a cheese factory, and in North Dakota all you need to do to break the law is lie down and fall asleep while wearing shoes!

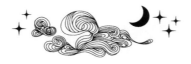

Artwork

```
I  L  L  U  S  T  R  A  T  I  O  N  K
B  A  R  G  R  E  L  I  E  F  Y  E  I
G  B  O  I  S  M  E  F  V  K  A  H  T
V  R  H  V  K  P  N  I  S  E  R  W  A
C  B  A  N  E  E  S  F  A  X  A  P  B
H  A  E  D  M  R  L  P  W  S  U  H  E
L  S  R  A  A  A  L  P  H  L  A  O  P
O  E  W  I  R  T  O  A  V  V  H  T  N
O  N  S  U  C  R  I  R  Y  M  T  O  A
H  I  M  A  I  A  W  O  W  E  O  G  N
C  L  Y  G  E  D  T  L  N  T  F  R  P
S  F  A  A  C  B  P  U  R  L  F  A  L
C  M  D  A  W  W  B  A  R  O  P  P  P
I  S  H  A  H  V  C  M  S  E  H  H  E
V  E  Z  A  L  G  P  U  R  R  E  Y  S
```

BATIK	ILLUSTRATION	PHOTOGRAPHY
CARICATURE	LINES	RELIEF
CARTOON	MURAL	RESIN
EASEL	ORIGAMI	SCHOOL
GLAZE	OVERLAY	TEMPERA
GRADATION	PAPER	WASH

"It is no small art to sleep: for that purpose you must keep awake all day."

Friedrich Nietzsche

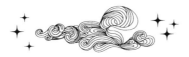

Diary

```
B A G E I P L A N E I O S
R E C O R D E C B M Y L V
S A T G G P V A G F E P N
W M D T R Y A D W E S H S
T U M N S A R E P D G S E
L S Y P E P T M R N E N R
A I T R C G Y I R N I J V
C N N F R T A C T L O G E
T G U U E T F I N U F E R
I S O E T B W O R N D M A
V D C S E E M N O R E E V
I I C H Y I A P B D H F G
T A A E T L E T R C N I B
Y R B T C H R O N I C L E
N Y S A F U D C A M F L E
```

ACADEMIC	DREAM	ONLINE
ACCOUNT	EYEWITNESS	PEPYS
ACTIVITY	FOOD	RECORD
AGENDA	GRATITUDE	SECRET
CHRONICLE	JOURNAL	SLEEP
DIARY	MUSINGS	TRAVEL

Sleep tip—Keep a sleep diary:

A sleep diary might help you to see patterns in habits or activities that are impacting your quality of sleep.

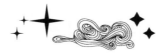

Moons of the Solar System

```
M  A  N  H  A  U  E  N  X  V  P  L  F
N  A  T  I  T  E  A  N  C  L  E  D  A
M  U  T  N  O  R  E  B  O  U  I  J  S
N  E  E  L  P  L  O  U  T  I  P  F  I
E  L  I  E  K  M  E  R  R  H  D  I  H
M  V  L  N  D  W  O  T  L  O  Y  K  D
E  Q  U  L  V  E  I  F  L  I  P  C  U
X  K  J  E  S  K  M  E  J  L  B  A  B
A  I  Y  A  K  V  I  Y  L  P  E  R  Y
C  H  L  L  D  R  I  T  N  I  S  U  P
N  T  S  L  A  J  P  N  E  A  K  M  S
A  A  V  U  Y  K  A  R  F  T  G  E  R
I  K  S  N  W  S  R  A  P  T  H  W  U
B  S  I  A  R  N  A  Q  J  U  Z  Y  G
A  E  H  R  Q  U  E  N  E  N  E  B  S
```

ARIEL	GANYMEDE	OBERON
ATLAS	JULIET	RHEA
BIANCA	KALYKE	SIARNAQ
CUPID	LEDA	SKATHI
DIONE	LUNA	TETHYS
EUROPA	MNEME	TITAN

"The timely dew of sleep, now falling, with soft, slumberous weight inclines my eyelids."

John Milton

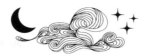

Greek Mythology

```
E S N M S A L W N R K I A
I C T O B M C S L I A F O
R Y M Y I N K H N S I A O
J L D E X R E G E A A I E
X L A C D S O C C R G T O
N A T U R E A H T Z O W B
A C U S D R A E Y F J N R
S Y H I G Z V R R D B M Q
I U P A T E O I E O R L I
D U E P O R E T S A B A O
S H A H S S E H I E M L I
O L A D P L T N C E M B R
R U S D D R T E L Y S A Z
O T A R E R O H C I S L N
E I J L G S E A N Y M P H
```

ACHERON	GRACES	ORION
ASTEROPE	HADES	ORPHEUS
BOREAS	HYDRA	PSYCHE
CHAOS	ICHOR	SCYLLA
ERATO	KING OEDIPUS	SEA NYMPH
GAIA	MEDEA	STYX

"Even sleepers are workers and collaborators on what goes on in the universe."

Heraclitus

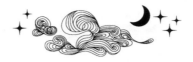

Friendly Words

```
Q E O B X S W B W Q N Z C
C I T M U H C O N E C F K
O B P A Q D L A O L F I R
N R S O M L D O Q R N G E
F E G B E P H Y E D C C N
E H H F R J L H R O V O T
D T O G U S S E H E C M R
E O L R G I D O H T R P A
R R W Z W S R G Z A O A P
A B Z L P T Y I I M N T F
T H L I L E J M B Y Y R P
E E R O Z R D A T A A I A
W I V O G E R E T L A O M
T E U Y Y V D E L P I T K
R W U D R B Z Y Y F I T F
```

ALLY	COHORT	KINDRED SPIRIT
ALTER EGO	COMPATRIOT	LOVER
AMIGO	CONFEDERATE	PARTNER
BROTHER	CRONY	PLAYMATE
BUDDY	FELLOW	SISTER
CHUM	HELPMATE	WELL-WISHER

"My candle burns at both ends;
It will not last the night;
But, ah, my foes, and, oh, my friends —
It gives a lovely light."

Edna St. Vincent Millay

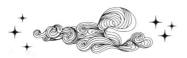

Occupations

```
K V B T A H W H R A X R D
R E K C O D R E C Z A O T
X U U L T R F B A R C T M
R N R A Z E M A S O N C Y
E O U B R E A A H J S O V
P I T E H N K Q I O T D T
E I E C N I Z X E D U A Y
E X O T A G T Q R J A N W
K F P R E N R U T C N H R
K W Z T Y E W P N P O E U
O N A O R L A W Y E R L D
O A W A Y I I T J A T K I
B T H O I V T C C U S E D
F B D E L I E I B B A R V
T O U D K C R Q N K V E V
```

ACTOR	CLOWN	POET
ASTRONAUT	DOCKER	RABBI
BOOKKEEPER	DOCTOR	REFEREE
CARER	LAWYER	TURNER
CASHIER	MAID	VET
CIVIL ENGINEER	MASON	WAITER

Sleep fact

Ensuring that workers were awake on time, particularly
in British industrial towns, was the job of a knocker-up
or knocker-upper. They'd tap at windows using a long
implement or less commonly a pea-shooter acting
as an alarm. This practice existed as late as 1952.

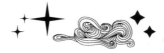

126 Words From the Letters in "HIBERNATE"

BEER   HERNIATE
BIRTH   HINT
EARTHEN   NEITHER
HAIRNET   RHEA
HEATER   TRIBE

```
B R E T A E H H T
T I B H A E H E E
H E R N I A T E N
A T E T H B A B R
E E H T H R R H I
H B T B T E I B A
R B I H E N H H H
R I E R T E I H E
I N N T T R R A I
```

127   Time to Wake Up

ALARM   MORNING
AWAKEN   ROUSE
BRIGHT   SHOWER
COFFEE   SNOOZE
DAWN   STIR

```
U D E E F F O C S
S A M D A B T G N
O C U R C N N R E
B R R S A I D S K
E R T O N L H A A
D I I R U O A F W
R A O G W S O A A
B M W E H T E Z S
P F R N O T B C E
```

> "The amount of sleep required by the average person is five minutes more."
>
> *Wilson Mizner*

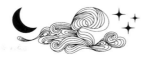

To Sleep
William Wordsworth

```
B E L O N G N I L L I W T
R D S N O I V I L B O T E
E E S D H G N I H S I W L
T L E E D E S A E L P R U
A I N E Y C L G O A E F V
W C K P B R E V F S E L I
E N E L E N E S H O V E R
M O E Y T P P K N E I S C
O C M L I A A C C A S M A
S E E E R F E T O O H I P
E R U T A E R C I Y M H T
R S C B E G U I L E D R I
I L U F T E R F A R N H V
T S G N I L K N I W T C E
S S O R C C H I L D O V E
```

O gentle Sleep! do they belong to thee,
These twinklings of oblivion? Thou dost love
To sit in meekness, like the brooding Dove,
A Captive never wishing to be free.
This tiresome night, O Sleep! thou art to me
A Fly, that up and down himself doth shove
Upon a fretful rivulet, now above,
Now on the water vexed with mockery.
I have no pain that calls for patience, no;
Hence I am cross and peevish as a child:
And pleased by fits to have thee for my foe,
Yet ever willing to be reconciled:
O gentle Creature! do not use me so,
But once and deeply let me be beguiled!

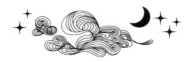

Curtains and Drapes

```
T  C  I  L  L  I  R  F  E  S  T  Z  E
I  K  L  N  S  I  D  C  N  C  T  T  G
B  O  Z  T  R  Y  F  O  I  S  A  F  A
N  H  E  I  X  V  O  D  K  R  I  L  T
Q  N  J  K  S  T  V  Z  X  X  B  S  S
H  V  K  K  S  V  N  W  T  E  M  A  F
I  N  O  E  X  J  V  U  K  A  J  P  F
F  O  F  O  W  A  R  N  T  S  E  B  X
H  T  K  J  L  E  R  E  I  T  R  O  P
H  T  I  A  S  E  R  R  H  D  J  Z  O
Q  O  N  B  T  I  A  E  T  E  M  T  N
N  C  H  T  A  I  R  R  R  N  W  N  W
E  P  A  L  L  M  A  Z  F  I  L  I  V
U  P  Q  S  A  C  Z  B  D  L  Y  H  C
R  C  Q  L  K  Z  N  Z  G  C  B  C  X
```

CHINTZ	HOOKS	PORTIERE
COTTON	LACE	RAILS
FABRIC	LINED	STAGE
FESTOONS	MATERIAL	THERMAL
FIXTURES	NETS	TRACK
FRILL	PATTERN	VALANCE

"Twilight drops her curtain down, and pins it with a star."

L.M. Montgomery

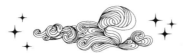

Making a List

To help declutter your mind and prepare your body for a sound sleep make a list of all of the worries, anxieties, and upcoming tasks that are occupying your thoughts. By writing down our worries we can relax, knowing that everything we need to think about is recorded and won't be forgotten come morning.

For example, right down any upcoming appointments you are worried you may forget, or list chores you wish to complete the next day.

....

....

....

....

....

....

....

....

....

....

....

....

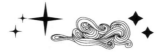

Modes of Transport

```
E G R A B U S A M E L P R
C T N B I C Y C L E I U E
E A R C H S A F P H E P T
C S R A U R H L S D E A P
B P W R I C A R O L V O O
A P B O I N I N A I D T C
Y U E W E A K A O A F O I
C I T B A E G R Y E Y L
I F X O Y O R E B O R L E
V F D A M D P P B N R M H
T L E T T O I P R O Y Y E
R S E Y A W B U S M S C S
U L N M G O C I C U U R R
C I D L A M A G L E V M O
K O A V H C S I O E B P H
```

AIRSHIP	DONKEY	PLANE
AUTOMOBILE	FERRY	ROWBOAT
BARGE	HELICOPTER	SUBWAY
BICYCLE	HORSE	TAXI
CAMEL	MAGLEV	TRAIN
CARRIAGE	MONORAIL	TRUCK

In our dreams—Departing:

This often indicates a breaking with habits or the
need to allow ourselves freedom and independence.

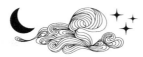

Wise Words

```
D R E T I N U E T U T S A
E O E E F A D T A N S G V
R R Y S C O N W F E L U T
O E E X P E R I E N C E D
T R A T I O N A L R X C C
U K B P P E N I G R H K K
T R A R J M I S E E B S N
G S A S I K O A I E H L O
I H F C P G S D A B R C W
S R A N D O H Y S W L L I
M M H L N L L T T I L E N
A F E A S O A I U G W V G
R B B E D U C A T E D E K
T L E A R N E D S I K R A
E T I D U R E I C E C E R
```

ASTUTE	KNOWING	SAPIENT
BRIGHT	LEARNED	SHARP
CLEVER	POLITIC	SHREWD
EDUCATED	RATIONAL	SMART
ERUDITE	REASONABLE	TUTORED
EXPERIENCED	RESPONSIBLE	WISDOM

"Never waste any time you
can spend sleeping."

Frank H. Knight

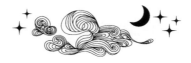

"HOUSE" Words

```
G L G B I M E E O N G H H
D A G G I A Q K S X Q P E
W K N H N Q A A A E C O S
F O U M N I C N K L T L U
P Q R L E E K S A K K A O
C L E K Q V F A J D W F M
G R N M D G R N E T F L Y
D U A E K R P F K R M K U
F I E F R E D L I U B H M
D H L S T T C L J O D X W
H C C Z T N Z R U Y Z X E
P L A N T I J N Z B M F Y
A K P L U A D K Q U I I K
Q D A F L P H K L W J F H
L Q D W O R R A P S E T K
```

BOUND	FLY	PAINTER
BREAKING	GUEST	PLANT
BUILDER	LEEKS	SNAKE
CALL	MAID	SPARROW
CLEANER	MATES	WIFE
CRAFT	MOUSE	WORK

In our dreams—Houses:

This is likely to reference our inner-selves,
and how we build our lives. The area of the house may
indicate the specific area of our soul that needs work.
Attic—memory, basement—suppressed emotions, etc.

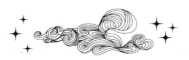

Astronomy

```
S O C R E S T E M K E R B
E T O B I N A R Y L A G K
P E S S R H I W B P E S T
E B M S U N E B U L A F K
N S I D A Y U T D T I R E
U H C I T H K J U H S A P
T C H O N J G R S U R C L
P H Y R E B N D N U T S E
E A T E C E E S R H H U R
N O I T A R R E B A I B N
S T M S H A O U S A C O G
T I R A P M A R U B O R N
A F O P L U T O B M M I E
R M D G A O R S H I E S I
S U N E V V A N I A T P F
```

ABERRATION
ALPHA
   CENTAURI
ASTEROID
BINARY
COMET
COSMIC

HUBBLE
KEPLER
MOON
NEBULA
NEPTUNE
ORBIT

PLUTO
RED SHIFT
SATURN
STARS
SUNS
VENUS

"You lose such a lot of time just sleeping!...
when you might be just living, you know. It
seems such a pity we can't live nights, too."

Eleanor H. Porter

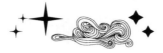

Dreams

```
Y F R I S A V M O T I E T
S Y P W E M M Y S H D N S
A E U D T U O C L H I I B
T R I M A E R D Y A D G A
N A R A P A A D U V R A I
A M S S U N O P I E I M C
F T L P O R Y E V V U I I
F H F I C U P E H E I S T
U G S R R G R L V O R V E
L I U A P I H S I W P N H
V N W T E Y B N E M O E P
D E L I R I U M G B C E O
Y P H O V S U I L F H R R
M N I N T R A N C E C F P
D I C U L D E L U S I O N
```

ASPIRATION	IDEA	REVERIE
DAYDREAM	IMAGINE	SLEEP
DELIRIUM	LUCID	TRANCE
DELUSION	NIGHTMARE	VISION
FANTASY	OMEN	VIVID
HOPE	PROPHETIC	WISH

Sleep fact

At least 95% of dreams are forgotten, unless they are particularly bizarre, or vivid, or we wake and recall them immediately afterwards. This is due to the suppression of chemicals that convert short-term memories to long-term ones during REM sleep.

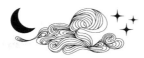

Loving Words

```
S  L  I  P  E  N  R  I  U  B  K  E  O
U  N  A  D  D  E  L  T  N  E  G  E  K
N  M  S  E  R  I  S  E  D  A  M  R  C
E  A  C  U  L  H  R  E  I  A  E  C  S
V  C  M  T  G  U  T  R  A  L  L  H  Y
B  V  N  I  S  A  R  M  A  S  B  E  O
K  P  N  A  A  A  R  T  D  D  A  R  K
I  E  E  N  M  E  I  E  N  R  I  I  H
T  R  L  K  A  O  L  C  N  N  A  S  O
T  E  L  H  N  I  R  B  T  K  U  H  R
E  A  C  S  G  S  N  I  A  R  I  U  X
N  B  H  H  E  H  M  E  C  I  O  S  S
V  I  T  C  L  A  O  B  I  M  M  Y  S
P  L  E  C  T  P  J  B  A  F  D  A  A
S  E  H  E  V  U  C  R  E  V  A  N  P
```

AMIABLE	DESIRE	RELATIONSHIP
AMOUR	GENTLE	ROMANCE
ANGEL	INTIMATE	SUGAR
CHERISH	KISS	TREASURE
CRUSH	KITTEN	VENUS
DELIGHT	MARRIAGE	YEARN

"I breathe slowly and deeply. I make my eyes still under eyelids, I make my mind still, and soon, Sleep, seeing a perfect reproduction of himself, comes to be united with his facsimile."

Audrey Niffenegger

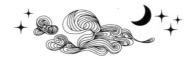

Puzzles

```
L O R U K A K E W H D I E
M A G I C S Q U A R E U R
N A N A G R A M S N U V A
S F T Y C I C I G O L C U
A L U H U R S F I H H R Q
U C I H E U O N J C B O S
K R D T B M A S R H G S N
O V R E H I A A T N D S I
D P R T V E E T U I H W T
U V L I W S R R I W C O A
C Y R E D I I L W C F R L
L T S R W K L S I G A D G
A I O A A Q U A R N O L A
C W Y B M G S U D O K U S
U G E R E D D A L D R O W
```

ACROSTIC	LATIN SQUARE	REBUS
ANAGRAM	LOGIC	SLITHERLINK
CALCUDOKU	MAGIC SQUARE	SUDOKU
CROSSWORD	MASYU	TRIVIA
JIGSAW	MATHEMATICAL	WORD LADDER
KAKURO	NURIKABE	WORDSEARCH

Sleep tip—Don't just lie there:

Trying to force yourself to sleep won't work, get up, try an activity—such as the puzzles in this book—and return to bed when you feel sleepier.

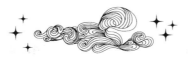

Sheep Breeds

```
N C T J T E N E B R A Y W
Y I U E C E N D B C U A M
E S X U A S T L A N E C R
L E T T M M M A O L H H B
L E M C B Y A O O C A E K
O V L H R R M H I T N V N
H A U A I O F N S N R I O
N M E G D R I R S A O O L
Y E B E G E C X R S M T S
G R F C E A I C W S A I E
T I L Y M U O R B E N S G
C N A Y Y T E B R U O U B
Y O L B T B D T T O V T I
S T S E R O F N U L C E P
F A V I O L A S E G E S U
```

ARCOTT	GUTE	OUESSANT
CAMBRIDGE	LINCOLN	ROMANOV
CHEVIOT	LLEYN	SOAY
CLUN FOREST	LONK	ST CROIX
CORRIEDALE	MASHAM	TEXEL
DALA	MERINO	TUNIS

"When I'm worried and I can't sleep
I count my blessings instead of sheep."

Irving Berlin

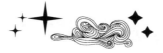

Birth Day

```
B R S H T N O M E N I N Y
L W A H S A U A U O C T W
U X Q E F I W D I M I J Y
Y S Q Q G I E N O N M R E
W R C Y Y L F L R C C X L
S B R A I A S E H T T A T
L G R V N P T F S U Y O N
D A E T E A U R C E J B R
B R R C M L I F T W I L V
Y B R U L F F T N R K W W
I O M T T A E B T R A E H
F Z E S T A X H D W Z I R
I R T H Q F N D S E R G F
M M E H D E H B M L W H J
I R E T N R O B W E N T D
```

BIRTH	FULL-TERM	NATURAL
DELIVERY	HEARTBEAT	NEWBORN
DOCTOR	INFANT	NINE MONTHS
FATHER	LAYETTE	SCAN
FIRST CRY	MATERNITY	SHAWL
FORCEPS	MIDWIFE	WEIGHT

In our dreams—Pregnancy:

This may indicate a long waiting period for something, such as finishing a project. Or an area of new potential opening up within ourselves.

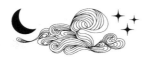

139   Words From the Letters in "SLUMBER"

ELMS   RULE
LEMUR   RUMBLE
LURE   SERUM
REBUS   UMBER
RUBS   USER

```
S  U  M  B  S  L  E  R  R
E  S  M  B  B  L  U  U  E
S  M  U  R  E  S  M  L  M
E  R  U  R  U  B  E  S  L
E  L  E  S  E  M  M  L  U
B  S  B  R  M  L  E  E  E
U  R  E  M  E  R  U  L  L
L  L  M  U  U  S  E  U  E
S  U  B  E  R  R  E  R  S
```

140   Under the Bed

BOOKS   SHOES
CATS   SOCKS
CLOTHES   STORAGE
LUGGAGE   TOYS
MONSTER   TRUNK

```
S  S  Y  S  F  O  R  O  E
K  R  E  Y  H  E  O  G  S
O  S  C  H  T  O  A  D  S
O  K  Y  S  T  G  E  T  T
B  U  N  O  G  O  A  S  E
E  O  S  U  T  C  L  O  R
M  A  L  E  R  F  G  C  A
L  I  D  E  H  T  E  K  G
D  E  G  A  R  O  T  S  E
```

"Sleep is like a cat: It only comes
to you if you ignore it."

Gillian Flynn

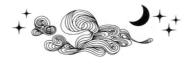

Active

```
X Y M P E Y C K P P J D Z
R D N D E F F I C I E N T
K Q E B D Q B P P V V W G
C R U T C U N R L Q F H S
X S O I O D A O I H M U D
Y I N W W O V M R S P U E
O A P L T N F P A P K D Y
M A D U I A U T L Y Z B O
K U I V S V L E H Q A L L
T G L A A G E L I G A F P
A N I M A T E D F T I A M
J I G P I Q S N I M B L E
Y V E Y K R P V T E D E M
B I N U B T R Y M S F R H
J L T D Q A Y T Y S C T N
```

AGILE	DILIGENT	MANIC
ALERT	EFFICIENT	NIMBLE
ANIMATED	EMPLOYED	PROMPT
AT WORK	INVOLVED	SPRY
BRISK	LIGHT-FOOTED	SUPPLE
BUSY	LIVING	VITAL

"Life is something to do when
you can't get to sleep."

Fran Lebowitz

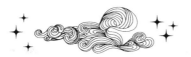

Dickens Characters

```
L  B  B  C  L  J  D  W  T  T  C  Q  C
D  I  E  B  X  V  N  Q  S  E  W  N  N
K  T  N  E  R  T  D  E  R  F  B  I  K
G  Z  E  G  N  E  K  C  W  B  F  G  W
I  E  A  A  H  I  D  B  A  T  R  A  O
R  R  N  X  M  K  T  R  A  A  D  F  P
P  C  O  S  O  Y  T  A  B  R  N  H  S
Y  S  O  Z  J  A  D  A  M  S  K  V  L
S  K  B  D  E  N  J  O  C  C  R  I  E
T  C  T  H  L  S  S  R  R  Q  E  R  S
E  N  L  A  Z  I  C  J  W  R  C  D  P
B  A  B  I  R  Y  N  Z  G  P  I  G  F
X  P  Z  E  L  T  A  H  O  G  K  T  B
R  E  D  L  A  W  A  T  I  S  G  K  G
M  I  T  Y  N  I  T  R  I  A  X  H  Y
```

ADAMS	FAGIN	REDLAW
AMY DORRIT	FRED TRENT	SMIKE
BARKIS	KENGE	TARTAR
BETSY PRIG	NANCY	TINY TIM
BITZER	PANCKS	TRABB
CODLIN	POTT	WOPSLE

"There is a drowsy state, between sleeping and waking, when you dream more in five minutes... than you would in five nights with your eyes fast closed."

Charles Dickens

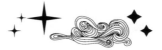

Trees and Shrubs

```
G A S U M A C V E C M B E
J E R I N T R O P C A L Y
E A C Y I S R E S L H S C
S G E A J A N D S A A L A
A D N A R A C A J D U D C
W L N A W O R E U W J A L
H R M O O R B J Q M L E F
I U S O R T V M V I Z R O
T K Y W N C A B L A K K S
E O R A L D E M H X C J I
B U R A M L E H C Y W D E
E N W A E U C C P S G U R
A V P M N T G R C A F A Y
M L O C I G X A T E A U A
E N S W S G E L S E L E O
```

ALMOND	LARCH	OSIER
BALSA	LEMON	ROWAN
BROOM	LILAC	SUMAC
CAROB	MAPLE	WHITEBEAM
JACARANDA	MEDLAR	WITCH HAZEL
JUDAS	ORANGE	WYCH-ELM

Sleep fact

Trees go to sleep too, research has shown they droop their leaves and branches at night by up to 10 cm and perk back up in the morning.

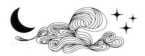

In the Air

```
E H O N D R I E R L S G L
T M A M A E T S E R A O J
S E E L B B U B C S C M A
U R E T P O C I L E H S O
D E I R N Y A M O V M O B
N E T A B E S D U A N U I
P O T S I M C T D W A N R
Q A I E N T A S S O T D D
H U R T A P A E G I E W S
A K A A U U E U M D U A U
Z E P S C L F R I A D V B
E W M K A H L R F R U E E
F G I M E N U O E U N S R
E T L N N E D T P P M A A
E C B R D A T C E N U E S
```

BIRDS
BLIMP
BUBBLE
CLOUDS
DUST
HAZE

HELICOPTER
KITE
MIST
PARACHUTE
PERFUME
POLLUTION

RADIO WAVES
SCENT
SMOG
SOUND WAVES
STEAM
WIND

"The twilight tints have left the sky,
and night commences her watch
over the world, high in the heavens is
her taper lit, around which will soon
glow a thousand kindred flames."

Henry James Slack

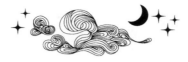

Journeys

```
S E N O I S R U C X E P E
B T A U L U U O A W I Y V
H A Y H G E D E P R T T I
R G P W Y V V T Y B G N R
S I E G A S S A P W N U D
W V R U O T Y N R G I A V
A A C E S Y V E A T S J L
N N H E R I I W L P S V W
D U U R S O V B F S O H T
E Q U I B O L L C I R S H
R A T L Y A I P K I C I W
L I W A W G D G X E K F V
U G G E H B Y M Y E R C Y
S E L T A L I A S A M T I
T N R U O J O S R A F C E
```

CROSSING	JAUNT	TOUR
DRIVE	NAVIGATE	TRAVEL
EXCURSION	PASSAGE	TREK
EXPLORE	QUEST	VISIT
FLIGHT	SAIL	VOYAGE
HIKE	SOJOURN	WANDERLUST

In our dreams—Journeys:

These are often related to how we carry out our day to day lives and how we move forward.

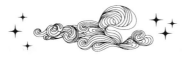

Sonnet 27
William Shakespeare

```
P  I  J  M  S  T  H  G  U  O  H  T  S
R  D  N  Y  E  Y  E  L  I  D  S  A  O
E  E  H  S  O  J  S  N  I  G  E  B  U
S  R  Z  E  A  L  O  U  S  B  M  I  L
E  I  Z  L  A  T  P  U  E  F  L  I  S
N  P  G  F  A  D  E  D  R  E  I  S  T
T  X  Z  H  N  B  R  I  V  N  E  N  Y
S  E  E  I  T  M  I  A  U  N  E  L  D
J  A  L  D  W  L  R  D  K  Q  T  Y  N
E  B  R  O  I  T  E  R  E  S  E  T  D
W  Y  R  A  E  W  A  S  A  T  H  N  K
E  K  P  W  O  D  A  H  S  G  E  E  C
L  O  O  K  I  N  G  A  I  T  A  C  A
S  Y  D  O  B  U  H  N  N  E  W  A  L
Z  N  D  R  O  O  P  I  N  G  E  F  B
```

Weary with toil, I haste me to my bed,
The dear repose for limbs with travel tired;
But then begins a journey in my head
To work my mind, when body's work's expired:
For then my thoughts—from far where I abide—
Intend a zealous pilgrimage to thee,
And keep my drooping eyelids open wide,
Looking on darkness which the blind do see:
Save that my soul's imaginary sight
Presents thy shadow to my sightless view,
Which, like a jewel hung in ghastly night,
Makes black night beauteous, and her old face new.
   Lo! thus, by day my limbs, by night my mind,
   For thee, and for myself, no quiet find.

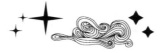

Lights

```
V K A I L X D N J N V C K
E Q T R E P S O L N O G M
F L A R E S P O R W O E A
W D A D C I O M V A O B N
T E Y O M R T E A D E V R
B T N K A O L M J K R E K
W C E E E Q I A M G I Y O
E A N R B P G L C L P L R
T R T R I Y H F E O F D E
L F O T E F T D P W A Z S
E E A I S T N J C S A W A
O R X I B A N O A L T A L
L S F B H P R A B B M A Z
M B U C V E H Z L E G I R
U I Y V E R V P L S R K G
```

BEAM	FLARES	REFRACTED
BLAZE	GLOW	SCONCE
BONFIRE	LANTERN	SPOTLIGHT
CHANDELIER	LASER	STAR
DAWN	MOON	TAPER
FLAME	NEON	WATTS

Sleep tip—Bright light:

Exposing yourself to sunlight first thing in the morning
can help to keep your sleep rhythms in check.

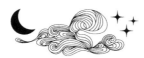

Poems

```
H S I F E H T A N S C L S
E I C I E I S M W A D A E
V A Y A D N E D L O G A V
R P P A R N A L V T D D L
E P E J K C E E O M N O O
D E C F I R R A E A V V W
N Z O R E B U S L E O G Y
O A E D E T T M I A Z H O
W M N A U C A S T L C G W
A I C M L E N H U R V F S
C H N T R O E A A A E E J
T E A D T P Q N M S U J R
E S H A I N A S L O U G H
S J L G W A N D E R R M E
S L E E V O L L I R P A R
```

A GOLDEN DAY   DREAM LAND   SLOUGH
AMERICA   LOVE IS NOT ALL   THE FISH
ANARCHY   MAZEPPA   THE PIG
APRIL LOVE   NATURE   TO AUTUMN
CINDERELLA   ROMANCE   WOLVES
DOVER BEACH   SILVER   WONDER

"Lie you easy, dream you light,
And sleep you fast for aye;
And luckier may you find the night
Than ever you found the day."

A.E. Housman

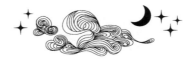

Dreams

```
S K Q A N K M D F S F E S
C S T A R D O M U O V H T
S Y C O E I L C B A O A E
M E W R P R C L L M L D R
O N R O O E U H E I D O U
T A D C S W G L E G U I T
H M H S R N D N I S N J U
E P T N I L S S Z A H C F
R F L T A T Y C K O F Q E
N N A S S N S E R X E L H
A E E L G V D A O P M S T
L M W A L N D G P O L E O
D O J U E I R Q N E F S N
L E V S Z D N E J P H G N
T E S E K S Y G K H M T V
```

ALIENS	HOME	STARDOM
CROWDS	LOVE	SUCCESS
EATING	MONEY	THE FUTURE
FAILURE	MOTHER	THE PAST
FALLING	NAKEDNESS	WEALTH
FOOD	RICHES	WORK

Sleep fact

Our brains cannot create faces in our dreams,
instead we dream only of faces we have seen in
waking life—even if just for a second. Most of us have
seen hundreds of thousands of faces in our lifetime,
giving our brains an endless cast to choose from.

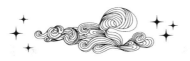

Decorating

```
H H S E M A I B D E R T A
S L A Z O M N N E A V R R
I S E F R I M E R U E C N
N F B H T X I N G P L T J
R R F E A I I J A L E G H
A S E A R N S P K E R A S
V S I D R G G C M A F N O
A N S Z D N A I G W A Z N
N C N O I A U S N L R P G
A G E N L N L D P G E M I
I E I I L G G D T H N D S
L L K D L Y E H C B I B E
S K I R T I N G B O A R D
E N G E F Y N I S I T E P
N R E T T A P G V A S G Y
```

CEILING
DESIGN
GLOSS
GLUE
HANGING
LADDER

LINING PAPER
MIXING
MORTAR
NAILS
PATTERN
PLANS

RAGS
SIZING
SKIRTING
  BOARD
STAINER
VARNISH
VINYL

"Spend money on your mattress
and bedding because these things
make a difference on your sleep
and, ultimately, your happiness."

Bobby Berk

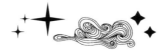

Stormy Weather

```
A L Q B W H T R U Y N Y Q
R H A I L S T O R M Z Y M
J M N R D L M G H E D I Q
D D O U U E S I E E Y U D
Y C Q N D L L R X M A N K
E B L Q S R B U G Q T V O
L S C O J O R A G I N G Y
Z M R I U G O A E E L Q
Z X S E S D Y N L V R S L
I N R Y W Q B T E O R Y X
R Z G O T O U U S N O N J
D Y T S U G H A R I T M S
R Q Q I H G F S L S M T Y
Y R E D N U H T Y L T N S
X P C N H D R D F A Y K V
```

BREEZY	GUSTY	ROUGH
CLOUDBURST	HAILSTORM	SHOWERS
DELUGE	HEAVY	SQUALLY
DRIZZLE	MISTY	THUNDERY
GALES	MONSOON	TORRENT
GLOOMY	RAGING	WINDY

In our dreams—Fog:

May indicate a confusion or unwillingness to confront things in waking life, and may go so far as to indicate an inability to even see the real issues we need to confront.

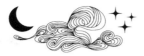

A New Bedtime Routine

Thinking about your current bedtime routine, based on your previous answers, map out an ideal routine below. Consider when you will stop eating and drinking, will you cut out certain items entirely or after a set time. Think about your daytime activity, when you will switch off from devices, whether you will include meditation, relaxing activities such as puzzles and reading, relaxing beauty treatments, list making, and anything else that you think might improve your sleep.

For example, "I will limit my screen time during the day, and cut it out completely one hour before bedtime".

....

....

....

....

....

....

....

....

....

....

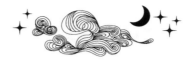

Late

```
B O R M U L E E E E T J N
O U T G O I N G O S A E H
U A C D D O E P A G L E U
N N R E G D S P E L Y Y E
P E S Y N C Y T A D L T P
U E B A D B I F Z T E R T
N L V L N E A R N L E P D
C I D E O S H E O V A E A
T H N D F Y C S I T T M A
U W I R O E B O I R S E C
A T H T R O U C A N D I K
L S E A M S E P O H I H H
S R B G E S E H E N S F E
N E R Y R D E U D R E V O
T C N U F E D L A T T E R
```

BEHIND	ERSTWHILE	OBSOLETE
BYGONE	FALLEN	OUTGOING
BYPAST	FINISHED	OVERDUE
DEFUNCT	FORMER	PREVIOUS
DELAYED	HISTORIC	RECENTLY
DEPARTED	LATTER	UNPUNCTUAL

In our dreams—Being late:

This may indicate a lack of attention to detail
or a feeling that time is running out.

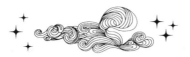

153   Words That Follow "NIGHT"

CLUBBING   MARE
DRESS   SHADE
GOWN   SHIRT
HAWK   STAND
LIFE   STICK

```
G N U E S P Y F L
K O A H D E F I L
W O W B D A S S F
A G B N C T H D E
H E A N I I R S R
A T T C R E I M A
S V K T S D A R M
C M L S C H E M H
G N I B B U L C A
```

154   Words From the Letters in "GLOOMIEST"

EGOTISM   MOOSE
GOOIEST   MOTEL
IGLOO   OSTIOLE
LEGS   SLIM
MILE   SMITE

```
I S S M S O O S E
G G O O O S S G T
L E E S T T O S G
O L O I M T E I I
O T O I I I O L E
G L L S O E T S E
E S M O I T O E E
I T G G G O I L I
M E L I M E O L O
```

"The longest way must have its close—the gloomiest night will wear on to a morning."

Harriet Beecher Stowe

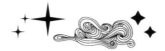

Medical Matters

```
E A F X C M L M Y B A E A
E L L B A I Q L G R A L M
S S E L E R A Q G N U L O
A U X X I N O L I T C Y O
E R O R G X O H S A X O R
S I R I A T A I T I I E G
I V N K T W F A A L H N N
D A L I D C R E O E N I I
D G S E I A E P T L V N T
E S D G C R S F M F S I I
D I Z T S R W L N U L U A
V S N T M K R D L I M Q W
D P S X I W N I R W B P L
Z E T E B A N D A G E B S
T S Y J W J A T S K V P T
```

ANGINA	FLEXOR	QUININE
AXILLA	GLOTTIS	SEPSIS
BANDAGE	INFECTIOUS	TESTS
CATARACT	INSULIN	THORAX
DISEASE	MUMPS	VIRUS
FISTULA	POLIO	WAITING ROOM

Sleep tip—Speak to your doctor:

If all else fails check in with a medical professional,
disrupted sleep doesn't have to be a part of your life.

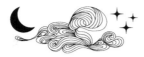

Poets

```
S O E R H W V H L M K U A
Q Y W U Z F M W E T X P W
P K L G S M C M I L L A N
Z S U O M R Y H D B R U H
E I H G J C I Q F K R E X
R S O A G G B X Z T L J B
O L K R K Y K W O E T T Q
Z L S T N E J D E K G R J
X O V Y E B S M S C A O R
H H Q S D I S P I Y A N X
P C B I S H O P E L H X T
L I L Y U A O E S A N U B
L N A H E B N G B F R E J
P R K R Y P U D A R L E Y
G V E P E X L V B S H A W
```

BEHAN	GRAY	MILNE
BISHOP	HULSE	NICHOLLS
BLAKE	KANT	NORTJE
DARLEY	KEES	PYE
EUSDEN	LEE	SHAKESPEARE
GOGARTY	MCMILLAN	SHAW

"And if tonight my soul may find
her peace in sleep, and sink in good
oblivion, and in the morning wake like
a new-opened flower, then I have been
dipped again in God, and new-created."

D.H. Lawrence

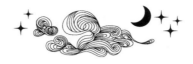

Root Vegetables

```
M A Y T R E S E D E N N S
P I N R U T J S U K O D N
O C A Y I I O R P O K T O
T A I D C M E L G H I U I
A S T A T E E B R C A N L
T S M U S P A C A N D G E
O A L L R E A I D U O I D
P V B O C M B R I S H P N
T A H U Y A E W S S P O A
E U C R R C I R H N I G D
E Y E L F D E R I W I M Y
W C H F R G O S E C M P U
S O F C N F I C H L I B C
K S S I N A M B K W E V E
C T G L E S T O R R A C S
```

BEET	DANDELION	PIGNUT
BURDOCK	DESERT YAM	RADISH
CARROT	GINGER	SUNCHOKE
CASSAVA	JICAMA	SWEET POTATO
CELERIAC	KOHLRABI	TURMERIC
DAIKON	PARSNIP	TURNIP

"God has made sleep to be a sponge by which to rub out fatigue. A man's roots are planted in night as in a soil."

Henry Ward Beecher

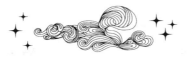

Wind

```
Y S G G F M Z A S N D F Y
D S E J O W J I G O C F T
E T N T L I V E D T S U D
T T T C N Y W A U K W P L
W O L B G F N I N P B X P
S V E T U R B U L E N C E
A S I R O C C O R Z D M V
N O R T H E R L Y G O N D
D N D T A B C A U O U Q M
S H H U Y I H A M D Z S R
T T L E C A L I M A O U T
O Q H X O Q S W E Y N T J
R M I U G F Q L I L D N E
M A G R Y H P E Z N A K U
Z A H B S W E M B I D G D
```

BLOW
CALIMA
DUST DEVIL
FOEHN
GALE
GENTLE

GUST
HIGH
NORTHERLY
PUFF
SANDSTORM
SIMOOM

SIROCCO
TAILWIND
TORNADO
TURBULENCE
ZEPHYR
ZONDA

"Sleep is when all unsorted stuff comes
as from a dustbin upset in a high wind."

William Golding

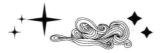

Lists

```
H W C E N T O N T I Y R B
D D I S T A A R V R B A R
E O L S W E A D A E G E E
I W C G H D W S S G R C T
N S Q K N L S N A D E A E
V F T E E O I T A E S R E
O C L O L T X S E L N R H
I A A G H B M E T R A A S
C S I N O W A S D F O S D
E E I E A E S T F N Y E A
N R A R S M P O E D I K E
S I Y I N G L I H M K J R
U E E I N L T A C W I N P
S S Z M I C O N T E N T S
K O O B G O L F F I R A T
```

ALMANAC	GLOSSARY	SERIES
BILL OF FARE	INDEX	SPREADSHEET
CALENDAR	INVOICE	TARIFF
CENSUS	LEDGER	TIMETABLE
CONTENTS	LOGBOOK	WHO'S WHO
DOCKET	RECIPE	WISH LIST

Sleep tip—Make a list:

You may lie awake at night with thoughts racing around your mind, by making a list right before bed, you will feel assured that you will remember everything the next day thus clearing your mind ready for sleep.

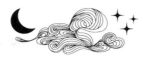

160   Words From the Letters in "DARKNESS"

AND   REND
ASKED   SEDAN
DANK   SNAKES
DRESS   SNARK
READS   SNEAK

```
S E R K K D S E S
S S K R A N S E S
E K N S E R A S A
R A S S S N K D E
D E K E E D D E K
E N N E D K A D D
A S K E D A A E D
K E E N K R N N R
S A A D E D R N S
```

161   Words Beginning With "STAR"

STARCH   STARK
STARDOM   STARLET
STARDUST   STARLIT
STARE   STARTLE
STARGAZE   STARVE

```
H S T A R T L E M
C T I L R A T S O
R A E E S L T T D
A R S L R A U A R
T D A T R A A R A
S U U V A A T T T
E S E S I R T S S
S T A R A R K S I
E Z A G R A T S U
```

"The darker the night, the brighter the stars."

Fyodor Dostoevsky

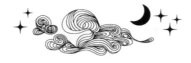

Fearless Females

```
Y H R D L D R I E D D T N
S B L M A L I N V V O I I
L T T N E R A D A B Y U L
M H A H H N U D A T S O K
F H S N G P I M O S Y L N
K M O I T I A E V O S E A
E U L C D O R Y T C G G R
L A S S I N N B E S A N F
L B R I D O E N L N H A S
E A Y H F O M V D A R M G
R R N P A S O E A C E B B
R T T M P R R W O C I U P
C O F G T S T V T R U T H
L N I R O G M H H A C I P
N O S N I K C I D L E R N
```

ALBRIGHT	DICKINSON	MURAD
ANDERSON	EARHART	OBAMA
ANGELOU	FRANKLIN	STANTON
ATWOOD	GOODALL	STEINEM
BARTON	KELLER	TRUTH
CAVENDISH	KHAN	TUBMAN

Sleep fact

Women are more likely to multitask during the day than men and as a result they need an average of 20 minutes more sleep—more brain activity in the day means more recovery time needed at night.

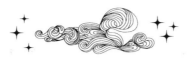

Capital Cities of the World

```
T W O H C A I R O T E R P
Y R E X L X F C E O O B S
T Q W I O A X M Q M S E W
I Y M G A A T G E B R L A
C A A B X D I L I I A T O
A M J O T H R X A S E A P
M O S A U L G S V L U B R
A U V C T N O A C A G A U
N S P T S N D S Y M A R A
A S T L E V K E R A R I Z
P O P U G N G Y K B P A U
X U B O Z W A D A A V M W
R K Y E R E V A N D B L L
F R H S O F I A O U O U O
U O Z R D A E T C R J B L
```

APIA	LIMA	ROME
BUENOS AIRES	OSLO	SEOUL
CONAKRY	PANAMA CITY	SOFIA
DILI	PRAGUE	YAMOUS-
ISLAMABAD	PRETORIA	SOUKRO
KABUL	RABAT	YAOUNDE
		YEREVAN

"And one by one the nights between
our separated cities are joined
to the night that unites us."

Pablo Neruda

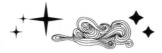

I wake and feel the fell of dark, not day
Gerard Manley Hopkins

H	G	U	O	D	S	S	E	N	T	I	W	E
H	O	U	R	S	E	L	F	Y	E	A	S	T
T	E	S	E	V	L	E	S	S	K	R	H	S
L	S	A	I	C	D	B	T	E	U	G	S	W
I	R	L	R	E	I	H	S	C	I	K	S	E
U	O	H	L	T	G	B	C	N	L	C	E	A
B	W	A	T	I	B	E	O	E	A	A	L	T
O	Y	E	L	K	R	U	U	N	M	L	T	I
E	R	L	A	F	I	C	R	N	E	B	N	N
E	S	E	S	L	M	D	G	N	N	S	U	G
T	P	T	I	E	M	Y	E	T	T	V	O	Z
S	S	T	G	S	E	A	E	C	N	G	C	G
A	Y	E	H	H	D	D	E	A	R	E	S	T
T	A	R	T	L	O	N	G	E	R	E	P	A
A	W	S	S	P	I	R	I	T	C	S	E	S

I <u>wake</u> and feel the fell of dark, not <u>day</u>.
What <u>hours</u>, O what <u>black</u> hours we have <u>spent</u>
This <u>night</u>! what <u>sights</u> you, heart, saw; <u>ways</u> you went!
And more must, in yet <u>longer</u> <u>light's</u> <u>delay</u>.
   With <u>witness</u> I <u>speak</u> this. But where I say
Hours I mean <u>years</u>, mean life. And my <u>lament</u>
Is cries <u>countless</u>, cries like dead <u>letters</u> sent
To <u>dearest</u> him that <u>lives</u> alas! away.

   I am gall, I am <u>heartburn</u>. God's most deep <u>decree</u>
<u>Bitter</u> would have me <u>taste</u>: my taste was me;
<u>Bones</u> <u>built</u> in me, <u>flesh</u> filled, blood <u>brimmed</u> the <u>curse</u>.
   <u>Selfyeast</u> of <u>spirit</u> a dull <u>dough</u> sours. I see
The lost are like this, and their <u>scourge</u> to be
As I am mine, their <u>sweating</u> <u>selves</u>; but <u>worse</u>.

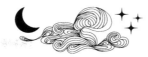

Mountains

```
E B A H G K T R A M S C A
K A O R E I A E S A N G H
I G G N E A R M S L N S M
P P Y A N F A O W U R C I
L A O R S U R Y J M U H S
L C S H L E A N U A A O T
E A I E T G E N U N M O A
F U O N G H N A L A U Y C
A C O N C A G U A S R U S
C M O G J F S N K L A U C
S G N E O H U Q A U P X A
M A R T I P F U M M Z T R
K A M E T G V E Y I A T M
U L R S N B E L B R U S E
S T E S T E O R V J B F L
```

ACONCAGUA
ARARAT
CARMEL
CHO OYU
EIGER
ELBRUS

GONGGA
JANNU
KAMET
KANGCHEN-
 JUNGA
KENYA
MAKALU

MANASLU
MONTE ROSA
NUPTSE
OLYMPUS
PARUMA
SCAFELL PIKE

In our dreams—Mountains:

These may represent obstacles we need to overcome.
Beginning the climb indicates facing our fears, and
reaching the top shows us achieving our goals.

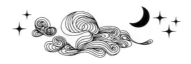

Romeo and Juliet

```
V C O U N T P A R I S W E
B T R E G N E S S E M N F
M L Y P A O W L V N I V D
O V H P A A E H U L F D S
T E M Y V C S M A P A T M
W R O P R W O S O G A P E
H O D U G I O I G R T C R
M N K N U R S E C B L C C
J A N I V O R R P E A G U
S U B E N V O L I O B I T
S P L I R S A F U O Y P I
B D N I S T M F W F T I O
E G F D E U G A T N O M P
P U Y I I T W M N Y F R B
E C N E R U A L R A I R F
```

BENVOLIO	KINSMAN	ROMEO
CAPULET	MERCUTIO	ROSALINE
COUNT PARIS	MESSENGER	STAR CROSS'D
DAGGER	MONTAGUE	TOMB
FRIAR LAURENCE	NURSE	TYBALT
JULIET	POISONING	VERONA

"Good night, good night! Parting is such sweet sorrow, that I shall say good night till it be morrow."

William Shakespeare

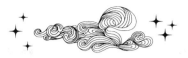

Eating Out

```
U N E M P D Y P S B P L U
Z O B M C E B K A E D C T
U Z E X L F C R G R N F I
N A D B I P C U J L T S C
L O A L A C A R T E I Y L
L T I R O L R V C L E R V
P L L T L K X O D M E A G
S I I I A E O D M E R R T
G B B R A V V I I A E A Y
I S O T G I R N Q T P H C
E I E F U L X E X A P S T
T R F S M R A R S S U I X
Y L P T O Y W S I E S F E
O C S E R F L A S M R S A
O G U Q C D R I N K S N A
```

A LA CARTE	EATERY	MENU
ALFRESCO	FISH	PARTY
BILL	GLASS	RESERVATION
CUTLERY	GRILL	SUPPER
DINER	MEAL	TABLE
DRINKS	MEAT	TAPAS

In our dreams—Food:
Food can represent the fulfilment of our needs
whether physical, mental, or spiritual. As such hunger
in a dream may represent an unfulfilled need.

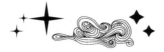

Watching the Night Sky

```
A F N H S F L P O A N S J
S A T U R N V O L G A P U
S I R E A G I D R N N P P
K E R N T V S R B I O L I
Y B T A S A A I U T O A T
M I E V L C R T R T M N E
A A L C U O A U F I V E R
P A E B A E P N E U U T D
O B S E R V A T O R Y S D
S M C E V S F R D P G O A
M S O E U I E R O E U A U
G T P N M E R C U R Y S B
N Y E U T R A C L O U D S
G V G S T E M O C H P A G
Y S R A M T S G T Y E M Y
```

AURORAE	MERCURY	SATURN
CANOPUS	MOON	SIRIUS
CLOUDS	OBSERVATORY	SKY MAP
COMETS	ORION	STARS
JUPITER	PLANETS	TELESCOPE
MARS	POLARIS	VENUS

"Sometimes at night I would sleep open-eyed underneath a sky dripping with stars. I was alive then."

Albert Camus

Solutions

1

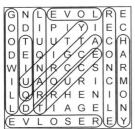

2

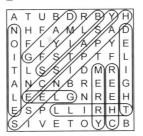

3

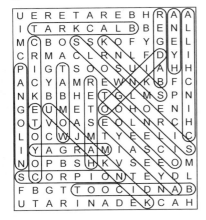

4

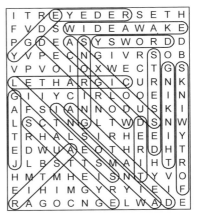

5

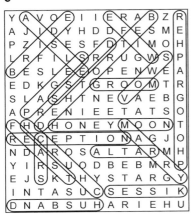

6

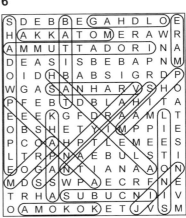

Solutions

7

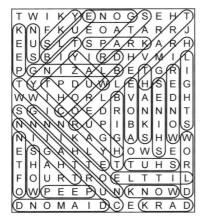

8

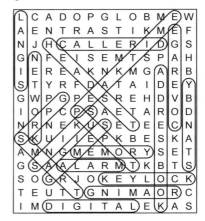

9

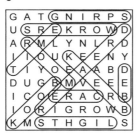

10

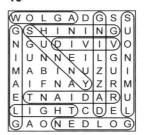

11

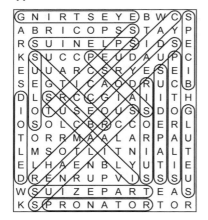

12

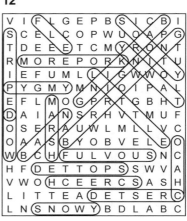

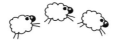

Solutions

13

```
S U I N O I T I U T S U A
C X D E Q O U A E C U N V
I O F O R L D S O O D A I
E S A C O U T U N T C M E
N T E C S S T H Z V A T
C T K A H R I C H S H S A
E E U G H B E I E I E T U
R E D T Q I C T G L N E D
S N O X O X Y H S L O R A
L I L A I R S E Z E Q X R
N M Y T E C A O Z Y M R G
G A C K H E S R Q D R E T
K X E Q T V T Y A U A U S
N E O D S T A T U T E S O
N L P R O C T O R S T U P
```

14

```
M L Y O M I L A H S E B E
P O T M D A A B A T A B H
I H R E O Y N H A Y E N F
A E A P C V S U R O H C S
T R U T H I G O L I A N E
S E Y P R E T R M N M I L
K B H A S E U L L N L A E
E U A V R V T S U T U S N
R S L O N D I S Z A O S E
B R Q F A I N T A N H H V
T L A A S Q E A P T L O U
F S U T H M H Y H E I A Y
N N M K R M H N N C L F D
V Y F V G I I A S A N E D
R V X E W S I M E T R A L
```

15

```
C H T H P A S V E G C D B
C U A I P L E E R O K I M
G J J Q O R B S L P S N E
E J A C T G H O T G H W E
S G W E F I N N Y C Y S K
E T B C N P E R I U T O H
H R O S U T E V M S S L N
A P N M C A A O P U S E O
M W E T A I T I D O M G O
U O F Z R C N C R O R E Y
I B O I I E H E D H A C F
L L O V N B L B C M Y P Y
I E T Y E G A O E L C E H
S A G E L I E X T A W A T
O L H S E S E R O P E R D
```

16

```
S R E D N U A S T
N I L L D S O T F
D V I L E N E S T
I E H K B N A O I
L R Y A R L M R D
L S L U N L Y O B
E L B H I L O I V
R Y O N G W M C T
L N A M L L U S A
```

17

```
A E L G G U R T S
E M E Y M C Y K O
E A D V O R I B S
L T L M F R B H F
E T B E M R R O E
M A U I U C A M U
T O S O E D W Y D
A H F H B B L E E
T E L I T S O H D
```

18

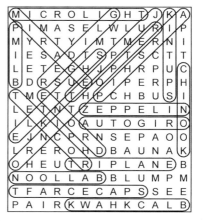

```
M I C R O L I G H T J K A
P I M A S E L W L U R I P
M Y R T Y I M T M E R N I
I E S A D T S P T S C T T
L E T E G H J P H R P U C
B D R S U E O I P E R P H
T M E T T H P C H B U S I
L E T N T Z E P P E L I N
I L K I O A U T O G I R O
E J N C P R N S E P A O O
L R E R O H D B A U N A K
O H E U T R I P L A N E B
N O O L L A B B L U M P M
T F A R C E C A P S S E E
P A I R K W A H K C A L B
```

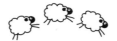

Solutions

19

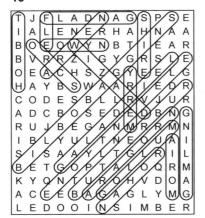

20

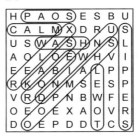

21

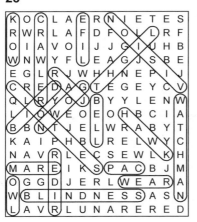

22

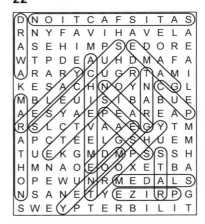

23

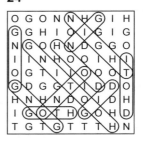

24

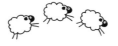

Solutions

25

```
L S L U S H D P N
C R P L V O S M S
A A W G G P E N H
E O R S D L I D S
S C V S U A B Y P
E U A U R N A N M
X Y I T V E B C U
O I U P S S G S B
F S T E K C I R C
```

26

```
L A Y G N O F R U A B E R
R E A E V E R N I R R Y C
N A V E R O K O C D E A M
U E B O I R K S M T D H L
L E S C F Y K C O D E O P
G E G S B S Q T A U Q S N
H M I E N I A G G N I A K
W A I G G I Y A H V Y H E
N E S A G E I Q E R E G S
A E R D L D U N A P O O L
M O V L H Y I O B L A P M
E O A H Z R H T U R C T E
O V R R T E E L A S O N R
A T R A N U S A N E R O R
H J K C R A R W B L O O M
```

27

```
N T H J M E L L I V L E M
I R C H A N D L E R V V F
A F V E M M H Y N Y U G I
W F F Y I C E E S D G L M
T P P L S H C S L T L N O
P S L D Y O D A B L A Y R
T E C L F G R P R M E E R
R V O N N E G U T K R I
H T G B G H O I P L H M S
I F R Z E R H C A D V Y O
S A T U R W Y W O Y I O N
D I C K I N S O N N G K I
F E S C A U O R E K N L E
Y G K C E B N I E T S O U
R R E N K L U A F A V O R
```

28

```
S O G W P W H A O R O G I
Y W N R L I G B T J N L H
R U I M U O L A W I U G S
T B B M Y N I A W W R D E
N A M C M R N O T U P J O
U R I Y E I R I G E U I U
O R L C N R N B N J S V M
C E C L H E Y G I G L E B
S O R I G I W T N U A C H
S U I N V R S P G B I N O
O W A G W U E R M D C A I
R I T T L A D U M R F D N
C F S F L S Z D H V Y Y G
K I C K B O X I N G Y O R
A R C A P A R I E O P A C
```

29

```
M E A H T N A M A S Y A L
K I B A B E C N C L E Y E
M I S S Y I S W U L D V R
U K T Y I K A L O L E D M
N K U T T I C K T Y Y O A R
T D A R Y K H D Q S B T R
R H E R A S L I S D M B M
I R L E S E E A S A I A
N Y D E I R S A C I S N L
I B V F I M C H V S I E A
S E R R W K E O U Y M A D
H A R N C S O E N T B R E
G R E S T T R O A A M B
S R G E S U O I C E R P C
I H R U M A E R A S Z O E
```

30

```
R R I U N R N S E
S N N R R E I N S
U I I U S E I I U N
S U E U R R N I I
U R U N N U E R R
S S U I I S S R E
E U N S U S I I U
R U E N S I R E N
N I S E S S N U R
```

Solutions

31

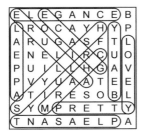

32

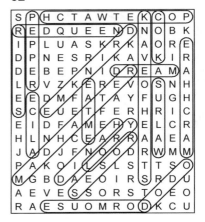

33

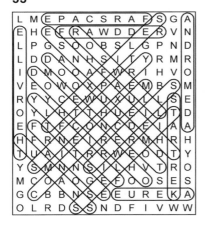

34

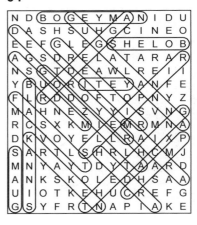

35

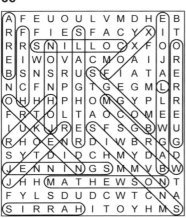

36

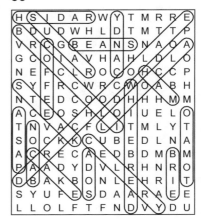

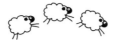

Solutions

37

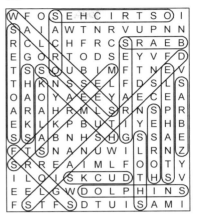

38

39

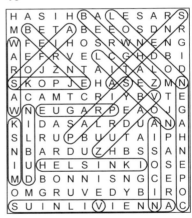

40

41

42

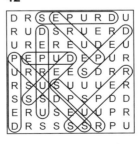

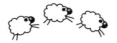

Solutions

43

```
U T M H S I N A V
T U Y O H V T A E
F O A Y D D S P H
R K L B E E A I E
B A E P S C E G Y
O E A I S C O R E
L R V E H O O E F
T B E P I O L N E
T H G I L F G E D
```

44

```
S E P L L E G L S
G I E I S N L S G
E S S E I N I L E
N P N L E N L I E
I L E E I E P P S
E E L L P E G G L
P P G I P L I G E
L I N E I P G I E
S E L I G S G N S
```

45

```
E H S I R E H C E
M M Y L I M A F M
F R I E N D V E P
N D E R E V E R S
A F F E C T I O N
L D H H S Z H N I
D I O E E U C A O
B A K R E G A R D
A U A E E Y C C V
```

46

```
S E R S E G N A R O S E R
E R A Y E K R U T G A G P
H S I F R L H A P S N P S
A Y S O T F E E A E A E E
S V I U H R A T G P N L O
T U N A O T P E T R A H T
U V S H A O N L L U B O A
N Y S P P L S I S N C N T
L R B C S G M M R E R E O
A A O D G A U O N S S Y P
W R E E E L E M N A E U T
N E C M P C C A N D A I E
S F Y P T Y O H I P S V E
C G A B D A C C I C G U W
E C I R N W O R B V Y W S
```

47

```
G H A V E O Y E H C I N B
I A V D R U N E C F N U S
G V U G N O V A L I S Y N
O P E T Y M G N T L D P R
G B U T I O L A E N E C U
U Y R S E E R E R G E H B
H A W T H O R N E R H R S
O S H E S K O K A E E R B
B E T Y B D I A C B U T N
S W W A C N B N A E L Y T
A C O L E R I D G E I H P
M T O V E K A L B U A T E
U M H T I D R A P O E L Y
D I T T T S N E S A F O G
L Y A D U H L A P S D E P
```

48

```
H M S B W L L A R T T A C
A G C D P Y T P A R X L T
L C O I L R A S S O U D C
I H U G M E T B U Y M I T
N G R A N T I W F O P S T
C B D E U A C F A A R S O
O D N G B S V E L I F P A
L K A F K A F A M W N E P
N G L A V B H Y O L E L P
A X R D E N G E N E D B L
B R A I I H D N R M Y Y E
O A G U O V M O O Y E L G
K M K B L N Y O E R V W A
O W H N P M G L A L N C T
V P P A R N E C N A C D E
```

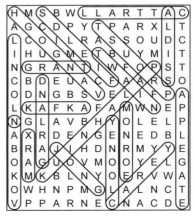

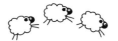

Solutions

49

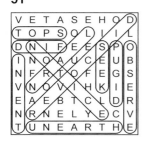

50

51

52

53

54

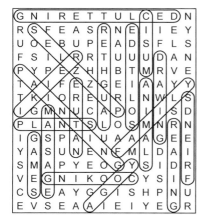

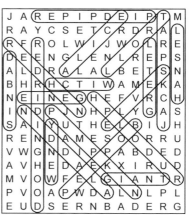

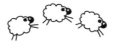

Solutions

55

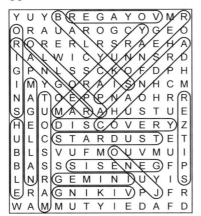

56

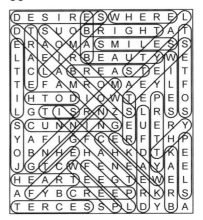

57

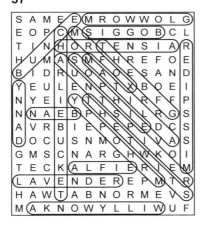

58

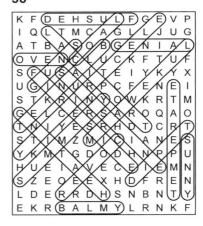

59

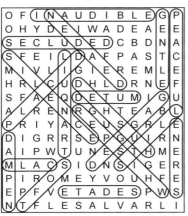

60

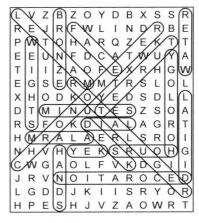

Solutions

61

62

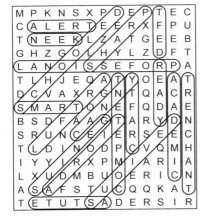

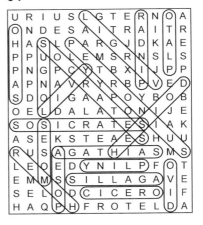

63

64

65

66

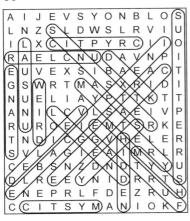

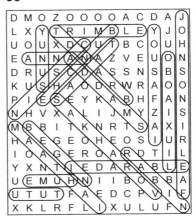

Solutions

67

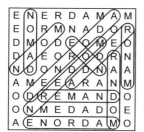

68

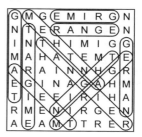

69

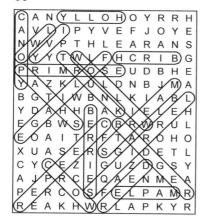

70

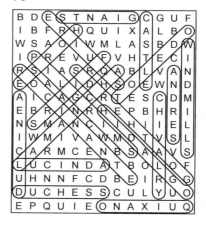

71

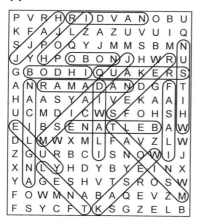

72

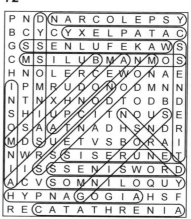

Solutions

73

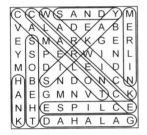

```
R R L A K L D L N Z C Q C
D V I C T O R I A M A R Y
G B U A U Y I R U J A N
L X Z E L T T R C L X Z E
E O E J D F H G S H I E R
T Z D A I G R R D K A T Z
I N W N E K A E E B G R E
H A Y E E G H R D D O D D
B M X Q Z T B A I I W R H
D I A X O E U E R A N N E
F X T I D J E N R O O B N
F Y Y M L I A D A L Z R
J W U H S L O M Q C O D Y
F N G K T D I H E L W A C
D E W D N D M W N S F E X
```

74

```
E T S E R T L T T
R P E I S U T S R
O A O E F S E E E
T F R T E R S R L
S C S R N E S E T
E E I U E N T S E
R A T R E S T N E
F O R E S T T I
T C I R T S E R W
```

75

```
C C W S A N D Y M
V A L A D E A B E
E S M A R K G E R
Y S P E R W I N L
M O D I L E I D I
H B S N D O N C N
A E G M N V T C K
N H E S P I L C E
K T D A H A L A G
```

76

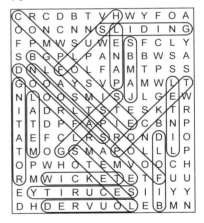

```
C R C D B T V H W Y F O A
O O N C N N S L I D I N G
F P M W S U W E S F C L Y
S B G P L P A N B B W S A
D N L E O L F A M T P S S
G O O A Y S V P A M W L T
N L O O S M I S J L G E W
I A D R L T S T E S K T R
T T D P F A P I E C B N P
A E F C L R S R O N D I O
T M O G S M A P O L L L P
O P W H O T E M V O O C H
R M W I C K E T E T F U U
E Y T I R U C E S I I Y Y
D H D E R V U O L E B M N
```

77

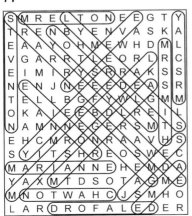

```
S M R E L T O N E E G T Y
T R E N B Y E N V A S K A
E A A Y O H M E W H D M L
V G A R R T L E O R L R C
E I M I R Y S R R A K S R
N E N J N E E E D E A S R
T E L L B G F Y W L G M M
O K A I E E B D L R E I L
N A M N N E G E R S M T S
E H C M R O N R A A V H S
S Y I T S H R E O S W E C
M A R I A N N E H E M D A
Y A X M T D S O T A G M E
M N O T W A H C J S M H O
L A R D R O F A L E E D E R
```

78

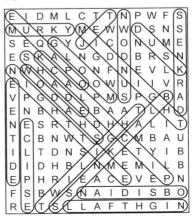

```
E I D M L C T T N P W F S
M U R K Y M E W W D S N S
S E Q G Y J I C O N U M E
E S K A L N G D D B R S N
N W H C P O N F N E V L K
E I O A A O W U I I V R
V P G D D L P M S P G B A
E N B H A E B A A T L H D
N E S R T H D H H A L I T
T C B N W T S G C M B A U
I L T D N S I K E T Y I B
D I D H B L N M E M I L L
E P H R I E A C E V E P N
F S B W S N A I D I S B O
R E T S L L A F T H G I N
```

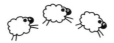

Solutions

79

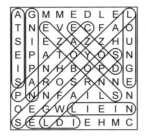

80

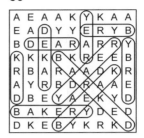

81

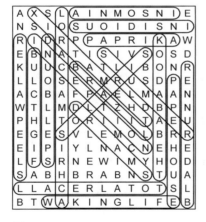

82

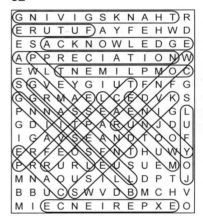

83

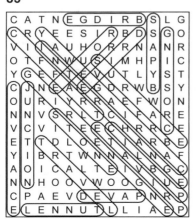

84

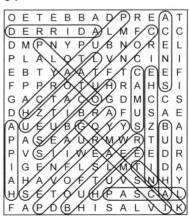

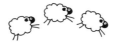

Solutions

85

86

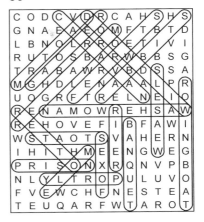

87

88

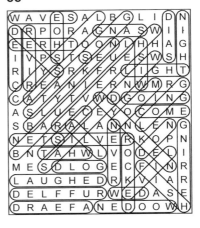

89

90

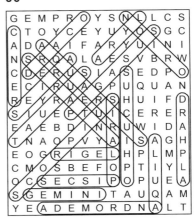

Solutions

91

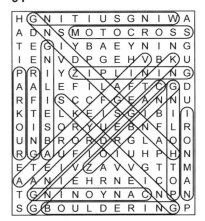

```
H G N I T I U S G N I W A
A D N S M O T O C R O S S
T E G I Y B A E Y N I N G
I E N V D P G E H V B K U
P R I Y Z I P L I N I N G
A A L E F I L A F T G D
R F I S C C F G E A N N U
K T E L K E I S G I B I I
O I S O R Y U E B N F L R
U N B R O R D R G L A O O
R G A U F I O I U H P H N
E T E I V Z A V V G T T M
A A N I E H R N E I C O A
T G N I N O Y N A C N P N
S G B O U L D E R I N G P
```

92

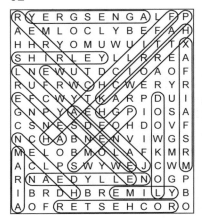

```
R Y E R G S E N G A L F P
A E M L O C L Y B E F A H
H H R Y O M U W U I T T X
S H I R L E Y L L R R E A
L N E W U T D C I O A O F
R U F R W C H C W E R Y R
E F C W Y T K A R P D U I
G N P Y A E H G P I O S A
C S N E S D E O H D O V F
N C H A B N E N V I W G S
M E L O B M O L A F K M R
A C L P S W Y W E J C W M
R N A E D Y L L E N O G P
I B R D H B R E M I L Y B
A O F R E T S E H C R O R O
```

93

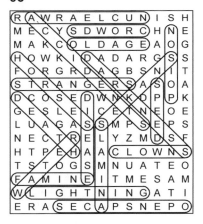

```
R A W R A E L C U N I S H
M E C Y S D W O R C H N E
M A K C O L D A G E A O G
H O W K I D A D A R G S S
F O R G R D A G B S N I I
S T R A N G E R S A S O A
D C O S E D W N K D P P K
G E S L E I C E T N F O E
L U A G A S S M P S E P S
N E C T R E L Y Z M D S F
H T P E H A A C L O W N S
T S T O G S M N U A T E O
F A M I N E I T M E S A M
W L I G H T N I N G A T I
E R A S E C A P S N E P O
```

94

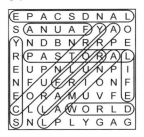

```
E P A C S D N A L
S A N U A F Y A O
Y N D B N R R P E
R P A S T O R A L
E U P N L U N P I
N F U F R I O N F
E O R A M U V F E
C L L A W O R L D
S N L P L Y G A G
```

95

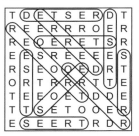

```
T D E T S E R D T
R E E R R R O E R
R E O E R E T S R
E E S R E E F E S
R S E O O E D R T
O R T R R R T T E
T E E O E T D D E
T T S E T O O E R
E S E E R T R D R
```

96

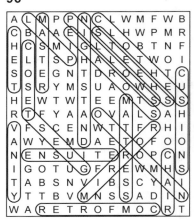

```
A L M P P N C L W M F W B
C B A A E I S L H W P M R
H C S M I G L T O B T N F
E L T S P H A L E T W O I
S O E G N T D R O E H T C
T S R Y M S U A O W H E U
H E W T W T E E M T S S S
R T F Y A A O V A L S A H
V F S C E N W T T F R H I
A W Y E M D A E T O F O O
N E N S U I T E R O P C N
I G O T U G F R E W M H S
T A B S N V I B S C Y A I
Y T T B V M N S S A D I N
W A R E T R O F M O C R T
```

Solutions

97

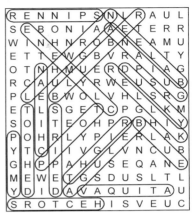

98

99

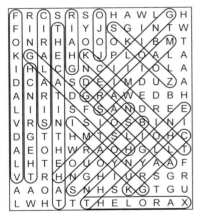

100

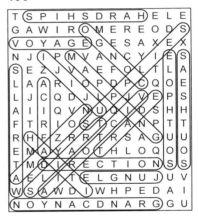

101

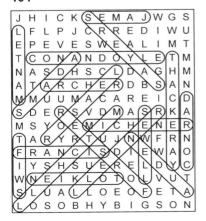

102

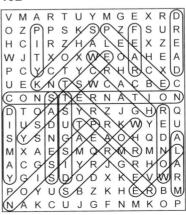

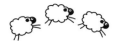

Solutions

103

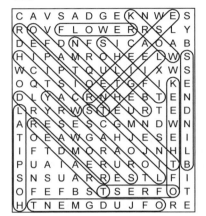

104

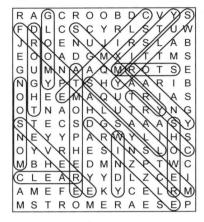

105

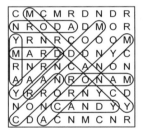

106

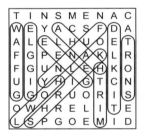

107

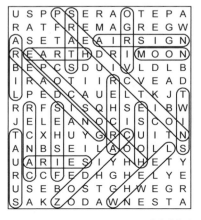

108

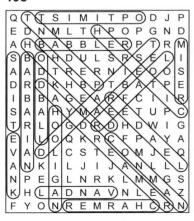

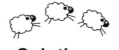

Solutions

109

```
E T A L O C O H C N P W J
B D T M I C J U T U H W S
G U L Y R E S T Z F Z J L
M G T N O I C Z Q C K E L
C N F T S L L A H E Y L E
I I R Q E E D I R N D L B
S C I T S R L M N O P Y H
U N E I D F A Q L X G I
M A D Z R U R L E V Q S I
I D O E R G R T I D I Q E
E T N F J X R F T E D E L
L Y I E A Y Z W K C S C S
S G O D T O H I N P U K H
G B N V F G N I H G U A L
D C S H C A E B E H T I B
```

110

```
E P E R C E M S D A S O N
B L G S I D E T I H W F I
A R H W F F R G R A N D E
U E O O Y U V A G N C U A
M B J A F R V O Y O R L R
G E W O N M L E S T D A E
A O M N H A C E M R T A D
R T A R N S T I A N R M
T S D L E E S N C P E M O
N H D R S B B O C P M S N
E T W R I W P F N A L T D
R A Q E F F I L C D A R C
L C B I L T W F W A C O E
S E U U E P R L T F D N W
R N W O L D A W F T V G F
```

111

```
S Y L L A S L Y P O O N S
A P R O I P H O S T O R D
Y D I B E E T H O V E N A
U L E K G N E P G I P T R
W L S E I E C E Y I A N
O A U E R U V E V L M D I
O B E C D F Y S H H V V L
D E F O Y R H U T I P I K
S S R Y M E N O O L M Y N
T A B V R C S L I N U S A
O B Y M C S E Y C T W C R
C S Y D I T E I C R A M F
K G L M N F G A R P A Y R
N A E J Y G G E P U E R A
B Y O N R E D E O R H C S
```

112

```
H D E L T T E S N U I H T
I P D I A L S I M M D N M
D R U E I U W A O I E S P
D E B Z P S B V O S R U E
E O T B Z H S B B S E N R
N C M N H L Y A T I H C P
I C O P E T E R N N T O L
N U V N W I A D F G E N E
V P A L F Y R F C E T S X
I I N T E U O Q A V N C E
S E I D N E S D S S U I D
I D S N S A R E H I R O S
B C H H O I A P D Y D U C
L R E B F R O O T L E S S
E H D T G N I R E D N A W
```

113

```
P A O T K B E S T I N G N
C P F C N E E D L E S U D
I P O N R G B S H P E S A
R L N F N E C I I M T A S
B I O C C I K L N M Q U O
A Q T R S O C R R D U G M
F U T S L R F P A H I I R
S E O S E V O L G M L N A
C R E D T N I H A S T V G
S O N G O I T R N Y E R N
E O T S I U T H G E E E O
W Y E T T F B C R E M R L
C E E A O R M L H E H U S
T R A P U N T O E E A B D
G G N I T S A B E T S D A
```

114

```
R E P E E L S Y A D N W M
V T D R I V E M A E O E I
D A H T S E P L E T I N V
S U P E R M A N R B C D M
N E M N O L L A F T I E A
A A G D B N E T S L P L N
N L M D N H E U L R S L O
I P G W Y A L I A S U G N
M D T M O R T D L Y S E T
A H H O E L I S Y O P E H
L O S D N O L A H U V U E
D O N F S G D O T N U E M
I A T O V D U E H W E H O
W H N U A U G E I H A A O
H G N B S L T O A E E S N
```

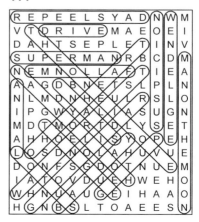

Solutions

115

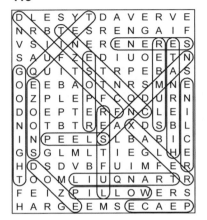

116

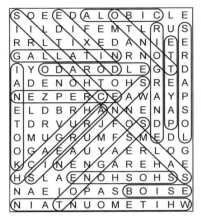

117

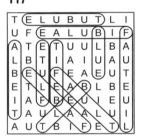

118

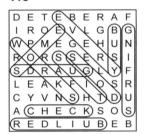

119

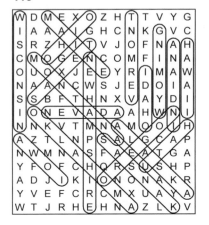

120

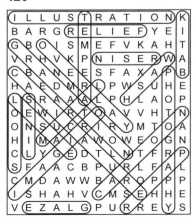

Solutions

121

122

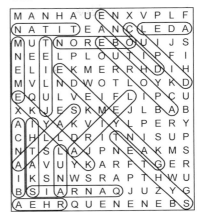

123

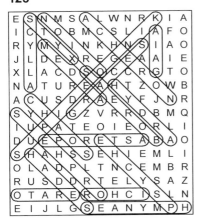

124

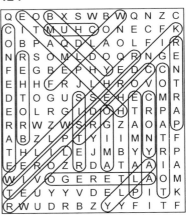

125

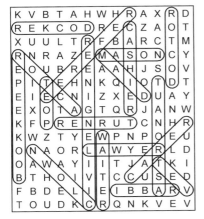

126

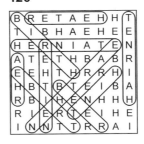

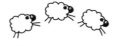

Solutions

127

128

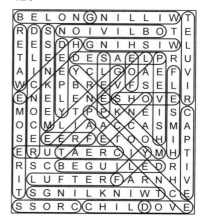

129

130

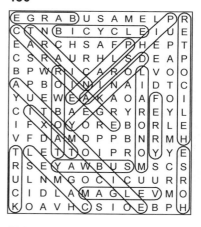

131

132

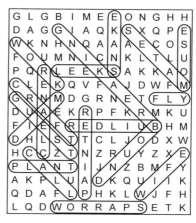

Solutions

133

```
S O C R E S T E M K E R B
E T O B I N A R Y L A G K
P E S S R H I W B P E S T
E B M S U N E B U L A F K
N S I D A Y U T D T I R E
U H C I T H K J U H S A P
T C H O N J G R S U R C L
P H Y R E B N D N U T S E
E A T E C E E S R H H U R
N O I T A R R E B A I B N
S T M S H A O U S A C O G
T I R A P M A R U B O R N
A F O P L U T O B M M I E
R M D G A O R S H I E S I
S U N E V V A N I A T P F
```

134

```
Y F R I S A V M O T I E T
S Y P W E M M Y S H D N S
A E U D T U O C L H I I B
T R I M A E R D Y A D G A
N A R A P A A D U V R A I
A M S S U N O P I E I M C
F T L P O R Y E V V U I I
F H F I C U P E H E I S T
U G S R R G R L V O R V E
L I U A P I H S I W P N H
V N W T E Y B N E M O E P
D E L I R I U M G B C E O
Y P H O V S U I L F H R R
M N I N T R A N C E C F P
D I C U L D E L U S I O N
```

135

```
S L I P E N R I U B K E O
U N A D D E L T N E G E K
N M S E R I S E D A M R C
E A C U L H R E I A E C S
V C M T G U T R A L L H Y
B V N I S A R M A S B E O
K P N A A A R T D D A R K
I E E N M E E N R I I H
T R L K A O L C N N A S O
T E L H N I R B T K U H R
E A C S G S N I A R I U X
N B H H E H M E C I O S S
V I T C U A O B I M M Y S
P L E C T P J B A F D A A
S E H E V U C R E V A N P
```

136

```
L O R U K A K E W H D I E
M A G I C S Q U A R E U R
N A N A G R A M S N U V A
S F T Y C I C I G O L C U
A L U H U R S F I H H R Q
U C I H E U O N J C B O S
K R D T B M A S R H G S N
O V R E H I A A T N D S I
D P R T V E E T U H W T A
U V L I W S R R I W C O L
C Y R E D I I L W C F R L
L T S R W K L S I G A D G
A I O A A Q U A R N O L A
C W Y B M G S U D O K U S
U G E R E D D A L D R O W
```

137

```
N C T J T E N E B R A Y W
Y I U E C E N D B C U A M
E S X U A S T L A N E C R
L E T T M M M A O L H H B
L E M C B Y A Q O C A E K
O V L H R R M H I T N V N
H A U A I O F N S N R I O
N M E G D R I R S A O O L
Y E B E G E C X R S M T S
G R F C E A I C W S A I E
T I L Y M U O R B E N S C
C N A Y Y T E B R U O U B
Y O L B T B D T T O V T I
S T S E R O F N U L C E P
F A V I O L A S E G E S U
```

138

```
B R S H T N O M E N I N Y
L W A H S A U A U O C T W
U X Q E F I W D I M I J Y
Y S Q Q G I E N O N M R E
W R C Y Y L F L R C C X L
S B R A I A S E H T T A T
L G R V N P T F S U Y O N
D A E T E A U R C E J B R
B R R C M L I F T W I L V
Y B R U L E F T N R K W W
I O M T T A E B T R A E H
F Z E S T A X H D W Z I R
I R T H Q F N D S E R G F
M M E H D E H B M L W H J
I R E T N R O B W E N T D
```

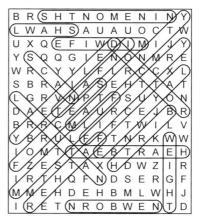

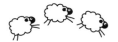

Solutions

139

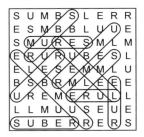

140

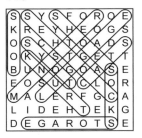

141

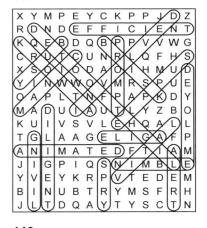

142

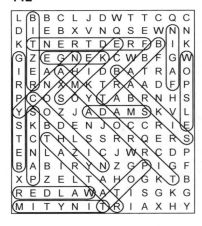

143

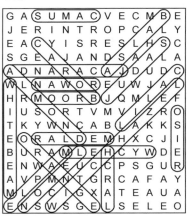

144

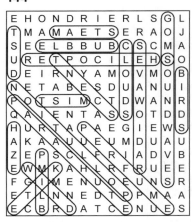

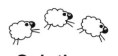

Solutions

145

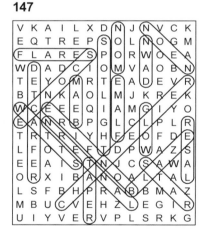

```
S E N O I S R U C X E P E
B T A U L U U O A W I Y V
H A Y H G E D E P R T T I
R G P W Y V V T Y B G N R
S I E G A S S A P W N U D
W V R U O T Y N R G I A V
A A C E S Y V E A T S J L
N N H E R I I W L P S V W
D U U R S O V B F S O H T
E Q U I B O L L C I R S H
R A T L Y A I P K I C I W
L I W A W G D G X E K F V
U G G E H B Y M Y E R C Y
S E L T A L I A S A M T I
T N R U O J O S R A F C E
```

146

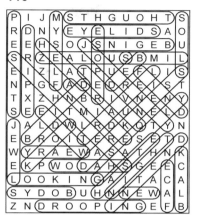

```
P I J M S T H G U O H T S
R D N Y E Y E L I D S A O
E E H S O J S N I G E B U
S R Z E A L O U S B M I L
E I Z L A T P U E F L I S
N P G F A D E D R E I S T
T X Z H N B R I V N E N Y
S E E I T M I A U N E L D
J A L D W L R D K Q T Y N
E B R O I T E R E S E T D
W Y R A E W A S A T H N K
E K P W O D A H S G E F E
L O O K I N G A I T A C A
S Y D O B U H N N E W A L
Z N D R O O P I N G E F B
```

147

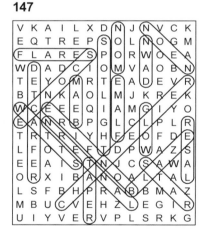

```
V K A I L X D N J N V C K
E Q T R E P S O L N O G M
F L A R E S P O R W O E A
W D A D C I O M V A O B N
T E Y O M R T E A D E V R
B T N K A O L M J K R E K
W C E E E Q I A M G I Y O
E A N R B P G L C L P L R
T R T R I Y H F E O F D E
L F O T E F T D P W A Z S
E E A I S T N J C S A W A
O R X I B A N O A L T A L
L S F B H P R A B B M A Z
M B U C V E H Z L E G I R
U I Y V E R V P L S R K G
```

148

```
H S I F E H T A N S C L S
E I C I E I S M W A D A E
V A Y A D N E D L O G A V
R P P A R N A L V T D D L
E P E J K C E E O M N O O
D E C F I R R A E A V V W
N Z O R E B U S L E O G Y
O A E D E T T M I A Z H O
W M N A U C A S T L C G W
A T C M L E N H U R V F S
C H N T R O E A A A E E J
T E A D T P Q N M S U J R
E S H A I N A S L O U G H
S J L G W A N D E R R M E
S L E E V O L L I R P A R
```

149

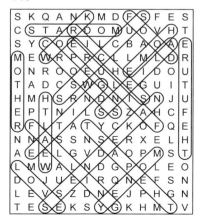

```
S K Q A N K M D F S F E S
C S T A R D O M U O V H T
S Y C O E I L C B A O A E
M E W R P R C L L M L D R
O N R O O E U H E I D O U
T A D C S W G L E G U I T
H M H S R N D N I S N J U
E P T N I L S S Z A H C F
R F I T A T Y C K O F Q E
N N A S S N S E R X E L H
A E E L G V D A O P M S T
L M W A L N D G P O L E O
D O J U E I R O N E F S N
L E V S Z D N E J P H G N
T E S E K S Y G K H M T V
```

150

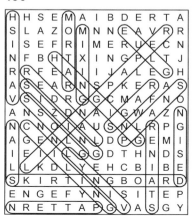

```
H H S E M A I B D E R T A
S L A Z O M N N E A V R R
I S E F R I M E R U E C N
N F B H T X I N G P L T J
R R F E A I I J A L E G H
A S E A R N S P K E R A S
V S I D R G G C M A F N O
A N S Z D N A I G W A Z N
N C N O I A U S N L R P G
A G E N L N L D P G E M I
I E I L G G D T H N D S S
L L K D L Y E H C B I B E
S K I R T I N G B O A R D
E N G E F Y N I S I T E P
N R E T T A P G V A S G Y
```

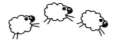

Solutions

151

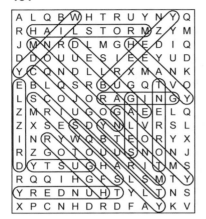

152

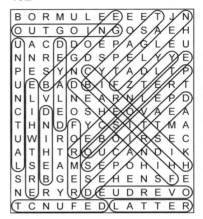

153

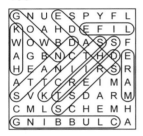

154

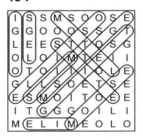

155

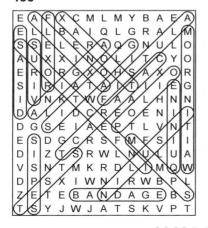

156

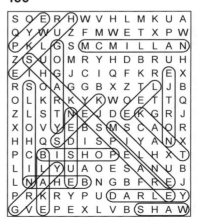

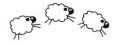

Solutions

157

```
M A Y T R E S E D E N N S
P I N R U T J S U K O D N
O C A Y I I O R P O K T O
T A I D C M E L G H I U I
A S T A T E E B R C A N L
T M U S P A C A N D G E
O A L L R E A I D U O I D
P V B O C M B R I S H P N
T A H U Y A E W S S P O A
E U C R R C I R H N I G D
E Y E L F D E R I W I M Y
W C H F R G O S E C M P U
S O F C N F I C H L I B C
K S S I N A M B K W E V E
C T G L E S T O R R A C S
```

158

```
Y S G G F M Z A S N D F Y
D S E J O W J I G O C F T
E T N T L I V E D T S U D
T T T C N Y W A U K W P L
W O L B G F N I N P B X P
S V E T U R B U L E N C E
A S I R O C C O R Z D M V
N O R T H E R L Y G O N D
D N D T A B C A U O U Q M
S H H U Y I H A M D Z S R
T T L E C A L I M A O U T
O Q H X O Q S W E Y N T J
R M I U G F Q L I L D N E
M A G R Y H P E Z N A K U
Z A H B S W E M B I D G D
```

159

```
H W C E N T O N T I Y R B
D D I S T A A R V R B A R
E O L S W E A D A E G E E
I W C G H D W S S G R C T
N S Q K N L S N A D E A E
V F T E E O I T A E S R E
O C L O L T X S E L N R H
I A A G H B M E T R A A S
C S I N O W A S D F O S D
E E I E A E S T F N Y E A
N R A R S M P O E D I K E
S I Y I N G L T H M K J R
U E E I N L T A C W I N P
S S Z M I C O N T E N T S
K O O B G O L F F I R A T
```

160

```
S E R K K D S E S
S S K R A N S E S
E K N S E R A S A
R A S S S N K D E
D E K E E D D E K
E N N E D K A D D
A S K E D A A E D
K E E N K R N N R
S A A D E D R N S
```

161

```
H S T A R T L E M
C T I L R A T S O
R A E S L T T D
A R S L R A U A R
T D A T R A A R A
S U U V A A T T T
E S E S I R T S S
S T A R A R K S I
E Z A G R A T S U
```

162

```
Y H R D L D R I E D D T N
S B L M A L I N V V O I I
L T T N E R A D A B Y U L
M H A H H N U D A T S O K
F H S N G P I M O S Y L N
K M O I T I A E V O S E A
E U L C D O R Y T C G N R
L A S S I N N B E S A N F
L B R I D O E N L N H A S
E A Y H F O M V D A R M G
R R N P A S O E A C E B B
R T T M P R R W O C I U P
C O F G T S T V T R U T H
L N I R O G M H H A C I P
N O S N I K C I D L E R N
```

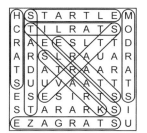
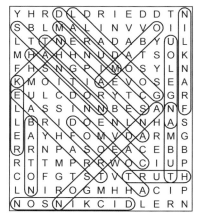

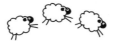

Solutions

163

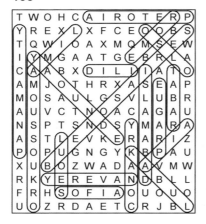

```
T W O H C A I R O T E R P
Y R E X L X F C E O O B S
T Q W I O A X M O M S E W
I I Y M G A A T G E B R L A
C A A B X D I L I A T O
A M J O T H R X A S E A P
M O S A U L G S V L U B R
A U V C T N O A C A G A U
N S P T S N D S Y M A R A
A S T L E V K E R A R I Z
P O P U G N Y K B P A U
X U B O Z W A D A A V M W
R K Y E R E V A N D B L L
F R H S O F I A O U O U Q
U O Z R D A E T C R J B L
```

164

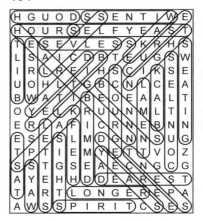

```
H G U O D S S E N T I W E
H O U R S E L F Y E A S T
T E S E V L E S S K R H S
L S A I C D B T E U G S W
I R L R E H S C I K S E
U O H L T G B C N L C E A
B W A T I B E O E A A L T
O Y E L K R U U N M L T I
E R L A F I C R N E B N N
E S E S L M D G N N S U G
T P T I E M Y E T T V O Z
S S T G S E A E C N G C G
A Y E H H D D E A R E S T
T A R T L O N G E R E P A
A W S S P I R I T C S E S
```

165

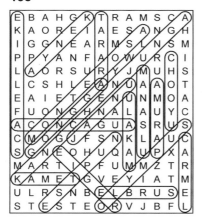

```
E B A H G K T R A M S C A
K A O R E I A E S A N G H
I G G N E A R M S L N S M
P P Y A N F A O W U R C I
L A O R S U R Y J M U H S
L C S H L E A N U A A O T
E A I E T G E N U N M O A
F U O N G H N A L A U Y C
A C O N C A G U A S R U S
C M O G J F S N K L A U C
S G N E O H U Q A U P X A
M A R T I P F U M M Z T R
K A M E T G V E Y I A T M
U L R S N B E L B R U S E
S T E S T E O R V J B F L
```

166

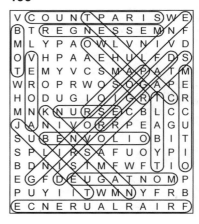

```
V C O U N T P A R I S W E
B T R E G N E S S E M N F
M L Y P A O W L V N I V D
O V H P A A E H U L F D S
T E M Y V C S M A P A T M
W R O P R W O S O C A P E
H O D U G I O I G R T C R
M N K N U R S E C B L C C
J A N I V O R R P E A G U
S U B E N V O L I O B I T
S P L I R S A F U O Y P I
B D N I S M F W F T I O
E G F D E U G A T N O M P
P U Y I I T W M N Y F R B
E C N E R U A L R A I R F
```

167

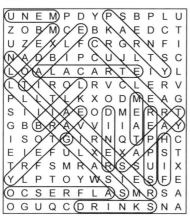

```
U N E M P D Y P S B P L U
Z O B M C E B K A E D C T
U Z E X L F C R G R N F I
N A D B I P C U J L T S C
L O A L A C A R T E I Y L
L T I R O L R V C L E R V
P L L T L K X O D M E A G
S I L I A E O D M E R R T
G B B R A V I I A E A Y
I S O T G I R N Q T P H C
E I E F U L X E X A P S T
T R F S M R A R S S U I X
Y L P T O Y W S E S F E
O C S E R F L A S M R S A
O G U Q C D R I N K S N A
```

168

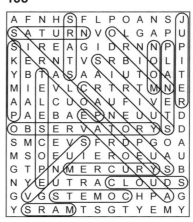

```
A F N H S F L P O A N S J
S A T U R N V O L G A P U
S I R E A G I D R N N P P
K E R N T V S R B I O L I
Y B T A S A A I U T O A T
M I E V L C R T R T M N E
A A L C U O A U F I V E R
P A E B A E P N E U U T D
O B S E R V A T O R Y S D
S M C E V S F R D P G O A
M S O E U I E R O E U A U
G T P N M E R C U R Y S B
N Y E U T R A C L O U D S
G V G S T E M O C H P A G
Y S R A M T S G T Y E M Y
```

Printed in the United States
By Bookmasters